MW00960642

The Complete DASH Diet and Exercise Blueprint for Weight Loss

A Comprehensive Guide to Combining a Low Sodium DASH Diet with Exercise for Optimal Results and Lifelong Fitness

Julia E. Chatwin, BSc

© Copyright 2023 Julia E. Chatwin - All rights reserved.

The information in this book may not be reproduced, duplicated, or transmitted without direct written permission from the author or the publisher. This book is copyright protected. It is only for personal use. You cannot amend, distribute, sell, or use any part or content within this book without the consent of the author or publisher.

This book is intended for educational and informational purposes only. It should not be construed as medical advice or a substitute for consultation with a qualified healthcare professional.

1st Edition 2023

All images licensed through depositphotos.com

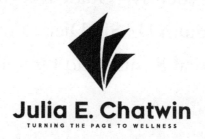

Julia E. Chatwin

TURNING THE PAGE TO WELLNESS

Table of Contents

Bonus Companion Books

All the trackers, logs and planners mentioned in this book are available free to download. There is also a free companion book which I have written called DASH Diet 30-Minute Workouts.

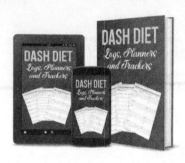 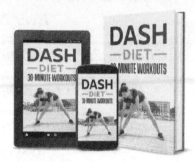

Also included is the must have "Weight Loss at Home" eBook. The accompanying Weight Loss at Home Cheat Sheet, full HD Video Course and Audiobook!

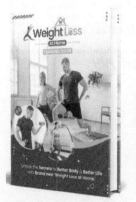 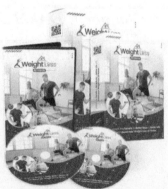

To get instant access to everything, please go to:

https://amitylifebooks.com/dashfree

Introduction

"There are six components of wellness: proper weight and diet, proper exercise, breaking the smoking habit, control of alcohol, stress management and periodic exams."

—*Kenneth H. Cooper*[1]

The urgency of tackling obesity, and the problems associated with being overweight, are more critical than ever. In 2016, the World Health Organization (WHO) provided a sobering statistic when they estimated that more than 1.9 billion adults were overweight. Of these people, they estimated that over 650 million were obese. Such data underscores the pressing need for a rational and evidence-based approach to weight loss and health management.

The cornerstone of effective weight management is a balanced diet paired with regular physical exercise. Both of these components have been substantiated by numerous scientific studies to be pivotal in attaining and maintaining optimal body weight.

Now, let's discuss a diet that really stands out; a diet that is recommended by nutritionists and healthcare professionals worldwide—the DASH (Dietary Approaches to Stop Hypertension) diet. The DASH diet was initially developed to lower blood pressure without the need for medication, but its myriad of benefits extends far beyond this objective. In fact, the

---

[1] Medical doctor, renowned for his groundbreaking research on the health benefits and improvements gained from regular aerobic exercise

DASH diet has been associated with a lower risk of several types of cancer. The reduced risk of heart disease, stroke, heart failure and diabetes has also been well documented. DASH has also been proven to aid in weight loss.

DASH emphasises the consumption of fruits, vegetables, whole grains, lean protein, and low-fat dairy products. The core principle of the DASH diet is not a focus on restriction, but on balancing nutrition and maintaining a long-term, sustainable, and healthy lifestyle. DASH does however encourage limiting foods that are high in saturated fats, such as fatty meats, full-fat dairy products and sugar-sweetened beverages and sweets

One of the major strengths of the DASH diet is its adaptability. DASH can be modified to suit individuals who wish to lose weight by reducing serving sizes, or pairing with regular physical activity. Whether you are a vegetarian, a vegan or an enthusiastic omnivore, DASH will work wonders for you.

About This Book (and why it's for you)

Embarking on a journey towards better health and weight loss can feel overwhelming at times. There are numerous diets, exercise programs, and conflicting advice that can leave you confused and uncertain. This book, combining the scientifically proven benefits of the DASH Diet and regular exercise, aims to cut through the noise and offers comprehensive, yet straightforward, practical advice.

This book, while rooted in the principles of the DASH diet like the first book in the series; "DASH Diet for Beginners", takes a different turn by focusing primarily on weight loss. Note that the first book was a comprehensive exploration of the DASH diet's impact on sodium intake and blood pressure control, diving into the specifics of how DASH can help in managing hypertension. In contrast, this new book approaches the DASH diet through the lens of weight management. It presents a fresh perspective, and straightforward strategies to shed excess pounds, while staying healthy. The book will still focus on the DASH diet principles, but from more of a bird's-eye view, allowing newcomers to easily grasp the basics while maintaining a strong focus on weight loss.

In essence, this book builds upon the foundations laid in the first, extending the potential benefits of DASH to a wider audience. You need not worry if you haven't delved into the previous book. This guide will provide enough understanding of the DASH diet to get you started on your weight loss journey. It offers a unique blend of dietary guidance, exercise advice, and practical tips that will empower you to reach your weight goals while fostering better overall health.

The book is divided into logical chapters, each addressing a unique aspect. While you're welcome to delve directly into a section that interests you, I hope that you will engage with the book in its entirety. In doing so, you will gain a comprehensive understanding of the transformative power of the DASH diet and exercise duo.

The **Weight Loss Primer** in chapter 1 sets the stage by providing a background on the science of weight loss. We will delve into its fundamental principles, debunk common weight loss myths, and provide practical strategies to set achievable goals. If you think you know all this already, think again. The biggest mistakes are made here.

Chapter 2, **Understanding the DASH Diet,** breaks down the principles of this heart-healthy diet, which, incidentally, was ranked as the best diet overall by the U.S. News & World Report, not just once, but eight years in a row! In this chapter we will look at potassium and its effectiveness in reducing hypertension. We will outline practical steps to adopt the diet, from grocery shopping tips to reading food labels. The process will be simplified, ensuring it is manageable and accessible, and certainly in no way overwhelming.

The chapter, **Exercise for Weight Loss** provides a comprehensive overview of the role of physical activity in weight loss and health. Different types of exercise, and how to safely begin your fitness journey will be explored. You will be guided through creating an exercise schedule that fits your lifestyle and goals. Whether you're a beginner, or an active individual looking to enhance your workouts, this section offers a variety of ideas and routines to help keep you motivated and challenged.

Combining the DASH Diet and Exercise presents strategies for integrating these two crucial components of weight loss. We will unravel the synergistic relationship between diet and exercise, aiming to help you strike a balance that works for you.

In **Staying the Course with DASH**, we address potential challenges you might face and provide strategies to stay motivated and consistent. We will look at addressing not just diet and exercise, but also the psychological and emotional facets of weight loss. Don't skip this!

In chapter 6, **Miscellaneous Tips, Tricks, Thoughts and Guidance** you are provided with a diverse collection of insights that bridge the gap between theory and practice. From time-saving hacks for those with hectic schedules, to nuanced suggestions for diet. It also offers a balanced perspective on popular trends like juicing and intermittent fasting within the context of the DASH diet.

Lastly, we come to my favourite part—the **DASH Diet Recipes**. Here, I have included all of the recipes mentioned throughout the book. Much thought went into these. They are simple to make and use easily sourced ingredients.

Our journey through this book will take us deep into the realms of nutritional science and exercise physiology, grounded in research, to provide a practical and effective blueprint for weight loss. It will be a journey not just about losing weight, but about gaining health, vigour, and a new perspective on a sustainable, wholesome lifestyle.

While this book contains a wealth of scientific information and practical advice, it's important to note that it is designed as a **simplified guide**, providing a general overview of the DASH diet and exercise for weight loss. The aim is not to overwhelm you with the minutiae but to offer a comprehensive, user-friendly manual to help kick-start your journey with DASH.

This book contains:

- Easy-to-understand language, making the diet more accessible and less daunting for beginners.

- A simple example 7-day exercise and meal plan to guide beginners on daily food choices.

- Detailed, but simplified explanations of the principles behind the DASH diet and how it contributes to weight loss and overall health.

- Practical tips for integrating the DASH diet into your daily life, such as how to dine out while sticking to the principles of DASH, and how to handle cravings and avoid high-sodium foods.

- Evidence-based information, including references to relevant research studies of interest.

- Recipes that are not only DASH-friendly but also easy to prepare and delicious. They can all be made with readily available ingredients and the book provides clear, step-by-step instructions.

So, if you are ready, let's get started on Chapter 1, which I hope you will agree is the only weight loss primer you will ever need.

One final note, if you don't understand a term or concept, please check the glossary. An explanation will most likely be there.

Frequently Asked Questions

I know you will have questions about the DASH diet and exercise and you simply can't wait to get into the book to find out the answers, so I've added some frequently asked questions here. Hopefully, this will satisfy your curiosity somewhat for now. Don't worry, these and other topics are covered in more detail later in the book.

Q. How does exercise complement the DASH diet in this blueprint?

Exercise, when combined with the DASH diet, not only speeds up weight loss but also helps in maintaining heart health, improving stamina, and building a strong mental foundation.

Q. Is it essential to follow a low-sodium variant of the DASH diet for weight loss?

No. While the DASH diet was originally developed to help individuals lower their blood pressure, it has evolved as a comprehensive dietary approach. It is beneficial for overall health, including weight management. While it's not strictly essential to follow a low-sodium variant of the DASH diet for weight loss alone, it is highly recommended! The reasons for which are covered in detail within the book.

Q. How beginner-friendly is this blueprint?

This book caters for individuals at all fitness levels. Whether you're a beginner or an advanced fitness enthusiast, the book provides a comprehensive approach to achieving and maintaining lifelong fitness.

Q. Are supplements like protein powders recommended in this guide?

No. The focus remains on deriving all of the essential nutrients from whole foods alone.

Q. How is this book different from other DASH diet books?

This book uniquely combines the DASH diet with a tailored exercise regimen, offering a holistic approach to weight loss. It addresses both dietary and physical activity aspects. It aims to provide you with the information you need to achieve optimal results.

Q. I have certain dietary restrictions/allergies. Can I still follow the DASH diet?

Absolutely! The DASH diet is versatile and can be adapted to fit various dietary needs.

Q. How soon can I expect to see results?

Results vary for individuals based on factors such as your starting weight, adherence to the diet, consistency in exercise, and your metabolic rate. However, many individuals will start seeing positive results within the first two to three weeks.

Chapter 1: The Only Weight Loss Primer You'll Ever Need

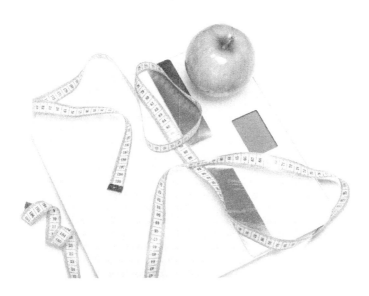

"Weight loss doesn't begin in the gym with a dumb bell; it starts in your head with a decision."

—*Toni Sorenson*[2]

Before we dive into the world of DASH, I felt it was important to provide this weight loss primer. It will arm you with the vital information you need before you start getting into the DASH specific sections of this book.

What are Calories Anyway?

Our bodies require energy (measured in calories) each day to maintain basic functions such as breathing, circulating blood,

---

[2] Bestselling author

regulating body temperature, cell growth, and supporting physical activity. This is referred to as Total Daily Energy Expenditure (TDEE).

From a scientific standpoint, weight gain is primarily the result of a caloric imbalance. This occurs when the intake of calories surpasses TDEE. Each calorie consumed serves as a unit of energy; when you ingest more than your body needs for daily functions and physical activities, the surplus is stored as fat. Over time, if you consistently consume more calories than your body uses, these fat stores increase, leading to weight gain.

However, if you consume fewer calories than your TDEE, an opposite state of caloric deficit occurs. Your body uses stored fat to make up for this energy deficit, leading to weight loss.

This principle, known as the 'energy balance theory of weight control', is supported by extensive research and unequivocal evidence.

While the concept seems simple, various factors influence both sides of the energy balance equation. These include your metabolic rate, the thermic effect of food, and even psychological aspects such as stress and sleep patterns. Achieving a healthy weight involves considering all these factors and adopting a balanced, sustainable approach to diet and exercise.

The 6 Basic Principles of Weight Loss

There are 6 basic principles of weight loss. Following these basic principles will help you lose weight safely and effectively.

- **Eat fewer calories than you use.** Or, in other words, use (or burn) more calories than you consume. This is the most important factor in losing weight. To be clear; in order to lose weight, you must create a calorie deficit—meaning you need to use more calories than you consume. To make it even easier to grasp—**EAT LESS** and **DO MORE!**

- **Focus on quality over quantity.** It's not just about how many calories you eat, but also the quality of those calories. Nutrient-rich foods will help 'fill you up' without a lot of 'empty calories' that do little to nourish the body.

- **Eat regularly.** Skipping meals willy-nilly will just make you more likely to overeat later. Eating regular, small meals, throughout the day, will help keep your hunger under control and make it easier to stick to your diet.

- **Drink plenty of water.** Staying hydrated is important for overall health, and it can also help with weight loss. Drinking water may also help you eat less, as water aids in the feeling of fullness. Water also helps in digestion, which contributes to weight-loss.

- **Avoid sugary drinks and unhealthy snacks.** Sugary drinks like soda and juice are often high in calories, which can lead to weight gain. Similarly, unhealthy snacks like chips or cookies are often high in calories and low in nutrients. Raiding the biscuit barrel will obviously make it more difficult to lose weight. It is much better to raid the fruit bowl!

- **Avoid fad diets.** Fad diets often promise quick results seemingly without requiring much effort. But these diets are often unhealthy and unsustainable, and they can actually lead to weight gain in the long run.

Sustainable weight loss takes time and patience. Therefore, focus on making small changes that you can stick with for the long term. It may only take two or three changes in your lifestyle to achieve this. They do not even need to be big changes.

Q. Why do we eat too much? Why do we eat 'bad' food?

There are several reasons why we may sometimes eat too much, i.e., consume too many calories. It could be because we're bored, or because we're stressed. Maybe we just really like the taste of certain foods. Whatever the reason, overeating can lead to weight gain, which can lead to a whole host of health problems.

Putting diet to one side for a moment—if you find that you're overeating on a regular basis, or eating food that you know is not good for you, it's important to figure out why. Once you know the reason, you can start to look for solutions. For example; if you eat when you're bored, try finding a hobby or activity that will keep you occupied. If you eat when you're stressed, try some relaxation techniques or talk to someone about what's bothering you. If you eat because you love the taste of certain foods, try to find healthier alternatives that are just as delicious. The scope of this topic is clearly not going to be covered in one paragraph, or indeed one chapter. This topic requires a whole book. Hopefully, though, this simple advice will resonate with you.

Overeating is a problem that many people struggle with, but it is possible to overcome. By taking the time to figure out why you overeat, and then making some changes in your lifestyle, you can start to get your eating under control.

There are also many reasons why we might eat "bad food", even though we know it isn't good for us. Sometimes, it's because we're busy and don't have time to prepare a healthy meal. Other times, it's because we're tired and crave comfort food. But there are also deeper psychological reasons why we might choose to eat unhealthy food. We might turn to food as a way to make ourselves feel better—even if it is only temporary.

If we're feeling sad, anxious, or stressed, we might reach for sugary, salty or fatty foods as a way to distract ourselves from how we're really feeling. This is often referred to as emotional eating. Of course, there are many other factors at play, including our genes, our environment, and our social circumstances. But understanding why we do it can help us to make better choices—and to break the cycle of unhealthy eating. Some people turn to food when they are struggling with mental health conditions, like depression or anxiety, in a hope that it will make them feel better. Whatever the reason, emotional eating is often a coping mechanism that provides temporary relief, but ultimately, makes the problem worse.

If any of this sounds familiar, there is a good chance that emotional eating is something you struggle with. Many factors can contribute to it and it is something that can affect anyone, at any time. Interestingly, research shows that women are more likely to eat emotionally than men. It is believed that societal pressures, hormonal differences, and various other psychological factors contribute to this gender disparity.

Knowing the difference between physical and emotional hunger is imperative when dealing with this issue. Physical hunger comes on gradually, and you rarely crave anything in particular. Emotional hunger comes on abruptly, often with cravings for specific foods like fries, chocolate or cake. It takes time to retrain your brain and go from simply grabbing food for a quick fix, to using healthy and alternative coping strategies.

If you find yourself frequently struggling with unhealthy eating patterns or believe you have a psychological issue related to food, it's essential to seek professional advice. Many people struggle with their relationship with food, and help is available. It's never too early, or too late, to seek support.

Q. Why is it difficult to lose weight? Or rather, why do some people find it difficult?

Well, there are many reasons! Here are just some of them:

- Our bodies maintain a certain weight. When attempting to shed unwanted pounds, your body might respond by decreasing its metabolic rate, or by heightening hunger levels.

- Losing weight requires making changes to diet and lifestyle. This can be hard to do, especially if you're used to eating unhealthy foods or used to being inactive. Change can be challenging!

18

- Losing weight requires time and patience and is not something that happens overnight—it takes a certain level of dedication and commitment to see results. This is true of almost anything in life.

Weight Loss vs Fat Loss — The Facts

When it comes to weight loss, there is a lot of confusion about what actually works and what doesn't. One of the most common misconceptions is that weight loss and fat loss are the same thing. However, they are actually two very different things indeed.

Weight loss simply refers to the total amount of weight that is lost. This includes both muscle mass and body fat. Fat loss, on the other hand, specifically refers to the loss of body fat. While you may lose some muscle mass along with body fat when you're trying to lose weight, the goal of fat loss is to specifically target and lose body fat. Losing muscle mass is not ideal and can lead to a decrease in metabolism. This makes it even more difficult to lose fat on future attempts, at least in the short term. Therefore, the focus should be on fat loss rather than just simply weight loss.

Additionally, when you lose weight too quickly, it's often mostly water weight or glycogen (stored carbohydrates) that you're losing, rather than body fat. If your goal is to lose fat and not just weight, then you should focus on strategies that will help you to achieve this. Some effective **fat loss strategies** include:

- Eating a healthy diet that includes plenty of protein, healthy fats, and fibre.

- Avoiding processed foods, sugary drinks, and refined carbs.

- Getting regular exercise. This should include both cardiovascular exercise and strength training.

- Intermittent fasting or strategic calorie restriction. We will touch upon intermittent fasting a little later on.

Weight Loss and Metabolism

When it comes to weight loss, a strategy that works for one person may not work for another. One of the most important things to understand is how **your own** metabolism works. Metabolism is the process by which your body converts food into energy. A high metabolism means that your body burns more calories, even at rest. A low metabolism means that your body burns fewer calories and is more likely to store fat.

There are several factors that affect your metabolism, but these are some of the most important:

- **Age:** Metabolism naturally slows down as you age. This is one reason why it can be harder to lose weight as you get older.

- **Genetics:** Your genes play a role in how fast your metabolism works. If your parents or grandparents had trouble losing weight, you may too.

- **Gender:** Women tend to have a slower metabolism than men.

- **Muscle mass:** Having more muscle mass can actually boost your metabolism. This is one reason why strength training is so important for weight loss.

- **Diet:** A high-protein diet has been shown to boost metabolism, while a diet high in refined carbs can slow it down.

- **Activity level:** The more active you are, the higher your metabolism will be. Even simple things like standing instead of sitting can help increase your metabolic rate.

Q. What happens to your body when you lose weight?

When you lose weight, your body undergoes several changes. These changes can be both positive and negative. It all depends on how much weight you lose, and how quickly you lose it. In the short-term, losing weight can lead to several health benefits. For example, it can lower your blood pressure, improve your cholesterol levels, and reduce your risk of type 2 diabetes. In the long-term, however, rapid and prolonged weight loss can cause several health problems. The message is clear—**slow and steady** weight loss over time is the better goal.

Q. When you're trying to lose weight, where does the weight loss occur first? This is a common question, and unfortunately, there is no easy answer. Where **you** will lose weight first depends on several factors, including your gender, body type, and how much weight you have to lose in the first place! But there are some general patterns that tend to hold true. For most people, the first place they will see weight loss is in the face and neck when you look in the mirror. Other places where you might see early weight loss include the chest, stomach, and legs. But again, this varies from person to person.

The best way to lose weight is to focus on healthy eating and exercise. The lifestyle changes presented in this book will help you lose weight all over your body, not just in one specific area.

Health Benefits of Weight Loss

It's no secret that being overweight can lead to a host of health problems. Here are some scientifically-backed **benefits of losing weight**:

- **Reduced risk of chronic diseases:** Weight loss, especially when combined with regular exercise, can significantly reduce the risk of chronic disease. This includes heart disease, high blood pressure, type 2 diabetes, and certain cancers.

- **Improved heart health:** Weight loss can lower cholesterol levels and blood pressure. This reduces strain on your heart, and decreases the risk of cardiovascular disease. Excess weight is one of the main risk factors for developing high cholesterol. Research has shown that even a small amount of weight loss can have a significant impact on cholesterol levels. One study, published in *Translational Behavioural Medicine*, found that people who lost 5%-10% of their body weight saw a significant reduction in fasting glucose, triglycerides, total cholesterol and LDL cholesterol. The study concluded that "improvement in risk factor status was significantly related to the degree of weight loss" (Brown et al., 2015).

- **Better sleep:** People who lose weight, especially if they were previously obese, often report improvement in sleep quality and duration, including fewer symptoms of sleep apnoea. This may be because extra fat tissue in the throat can block the airway. Although losing weight may help to improve sleep apnoea, it is not a cure. In fact, even people of normal weight can have sleep apnoea. If you think you might have sleep apnoea, talk to your doctor today.

- **Improved mobility and reduced joint pain:** Excess weight puts additional pressure on your joints, which can lead to pain and arthritis. Losing weight can alleviate this pressure, enhancing mobility and reducing discomfort.

- **Enhanced mood and mental health:** Weight loss can boost your mood, self-esteem, and overall outlook on life. It's also associated with a reduced risk of depression and anxiety.

- **Improved blood sugar control:** Weight loss can improve insulin resistance and help in managing type 2 diabetes.

- **Improved lung function:** Losing weight can lead to better respiratory efficiency, which can make physical activity and daily tasks easier.

- **Longer life expectancy:** Numerous studies have found a link between weight loss and reduced mortality risk, suggesting that maintaining a healthy weight could help you live longer.

- **Improved fertility:** Overweight and obesity can lead to hormonal imbalances and problems with ovulation in women, affecting fertility. Weight loss can improve these issues.

- **Increased energy:** Weight loss often comes with an increase in energy, making daily tasks and physical activities easier to accomplish.

Cellulite

Cellulite is a term used to describe the dimpled appearance of skin that is often seen on the thighs, hips, and buttocks. Cellulite is caused by fat cells that push up against the connective tissues underneath the skin, which results in 'puckering'. While it is not harmful, cellulite can become an unwanted feature of one's appearance. Many people find it difficult to get rid of.

The effect of weight loss on cellulite depends on several individual factors. However, in general, losing weight can help to reduce its appearance. This is because fat cells tend to make cellulite more visible, so by reducing the amount of fat in the body, you can also reduce the appearance of cellulite. Toning up the muscles under the skin can also help to minimise the appearance of cellulite. If you are hoping to get rid of cellulite through weight loss, it is important to focus not only on losing overall body fat, but also on toning the muscles under the affected areas.

Q. Will weight loss help with back pain?

The simple answer is yes, but there are a few things to keep in mind:

- Understand that carrying extra weight can put a strain on your back and spine. This can lead to pain, discomfort, and even injury. By losing weight, you are likely to reduce the amount of strain on your back.

- If your back pain is due to an underlying medical condition, such as obesity-related degenerative disc disease, then losing weight may help improve your symptoms. In fact, research has shown that even a small amount of weight loss (5-10% of body weight) can lead to significant improvements in back pain and function.

- Keep in mind that weight loss is not a quick fix for back pain. It may take some time for your symptoms to improve, but making healthy lifestyle changes is always a good idea—not just for your back, your knees and feet, but for your overall health.

- If you're trying to lose weight to relieve back pain, talk to your doctor or a registered dietitian first as there may be other underlying issues that need addressing.

Losing weight may help reduce the pain and other symptoms like sciatica. Sciatica is a condition that can be caused by a herniated disk, bone spur, or narrowing of the spinal canal, among other reasons. A common characteristic is a pain that radiates from your lower back down your leg. Losing weight may help relieve pressure on the sciatic nerve and improve your overall mobility.

Blood Pressure

It is well-known that being overweight or obese can lead to several health problems, including high blood pressure. So, it stands to reason that weight loss should help to lower blood pressure. Indeed, research has shown that even a modest amount of weight loss can have a positive impact on blood pressure.

For example, a research study published in the journal *Circulation*, focused on individuals who were obese and had hypertension. The study included 100 participants who were randomly divided into two groups; one group underwent bypass surgery while the other received treatment alone. After surgery, the study found that "51% of the patients submitted to gastric bypass showed remission of hypertension" (Schiavon et al., 2018). This demonstrates a connection between obesity and blood pressure, highlighting how weight loss can potentially contribute to its reduction.

Weight Loss Without Exercise?

Losing weight without exercising might sound too good to be true, but it is possible.

If you are really dead set on not exercising, dietary changes can work for you, but the results will be slower. Reducing calorie intake and making healthy food choices will promote long-term weight loss and maintenance. Cutting out sugary drinks and processed foods will also help reduce calorie intake, while increasing the intake of fresh fruits and vegetables will help provide the nutrients needed for healthy weight loss. Sleep and stress management are also important factors in losing weight without exercising. Getting enough sleep can help boost metabolism and reduce cravings, while managing stress can help prevent emotional eating.

With that said though, **combining** a reduction in calorie intake **with** regular exercise will **significantly** enhance your weight loss efforts! Not only can this dual approach help you lose weight faster, but it also brings numerous health benefits. Lowering calorie intake aids in reducing weight, while the physical activity helps burn extra calories, build muscle, and boost metabolism. Moreover, exercising regularly can improve heart health, bone density, mental health, and overall quality of life.

The answer is clear: implementing a balanced diet and regular exercise is a comprehensive and effective approach to weight loss and better health.

Tips on Getting Started

When it comes to getting started on your weight loss journey, commitment to adopting lifestyle changes is key. These tips will help you get started on the path to success:

- Reduce calorie intake by cutting back on high calorie foods like sweets, desserts, fried foods, and processed snacks. Conversely, focus on consuming fruits, vegetables, lean protein sources, and whole grains.

- Increase activity by incorporating movement into your daily routine throughout the day.

- Make it a habit to take a walk after your evening meal, or enjoy a bike ride at the weekends, or find a sport or hobby that involves activity.

- It's important to stay hydrated, so drink plenty of water throughout the day. Drinking water can help you feel satisfied and potentially reduce your calorie intake.

- To avoid weight gain, try to avoid eating at night. This will allow your body time to burn off those calories.

- Stay away from drinks like soda, juice and energy drinks as they add extra and unwanted calories to your diet. Water or unsweetened tea is a better choice.

- Keeping track of your progress is crucial in staying motivated and on track with your weight loss journey. Consider using a food journal or tracking app to monitor both your calorie intake and weight loss progress.

If you're finding it challenging to lose weight, and feel it is genuinely more challenging than it should be, consult with your doctor. They will be able to provide further guidance and support.

Progress takes time, but with dedication and perseverance, you'll be well on your way towards achieving your desired weight loss goals.

Start Meal Prepping Now

If you're looking for ways to stay on track with your eating habits while losing weight, meal prepping can be a game changer. By preparing meals or snacks in advance, you'll be giving yourself the best possible chance of consuming portion controlled meals while avoiding unhealthy choices. Meal prepping doesn't have to be complicated or time consuming; start small by prepping one meal or snack per day.

Once you establish a routine, you can gradually increase the quantity of food you cook. Planning and preparing meals in advance can be beneficial in terms of both time and money. By having prepped meals ready, you can avoid last-minute grocery store or restaurant visits. Additionally, when you prepare your meals, you have control over the ingredients and can steer clear of processed foods. If meal prepping is new to you, these tips will help:

- **Make a shopping list.** Once you know what you're going to eat, make a list of all the ingredients you will need. Never go grocery shopping when you're hungry! This leads to impulse buying and unhealthy food choices. If it's not on the list, you don't need it!
- **Prep your food.** Wash and chop fruits and vegetables in bulk, separate them all out into portion sizes ready for storing in the fridge. Measure out snacks ahead of time.
- **Store your food properly.** Store prepped food in airtight containers in the fridge or freezer.
- **Reheat (safely) or eat cold.** When you're ready to eat, simply reheat your meal or enjoy it cold.

Motivation and your Reason to Lose Weight

Weight loss motivation can be a challenge for many people. Having a compelling, personal reason for losing weight is paramount to success in your weight loss journey. This reason, often referred to as your 'why', acts as a motivation source and will help you stay focused and committed. This is particularly true during challenging times when progress seems slow or when temptations are high.

Your 'why' should be deeply personal. Some people want to lose weight for health-related reasons. For others, it might be about improving self-confidence, enhancing mood, or increasing energy levels. You may want to lose weight to be more active with your children or grandchildren, or perhaps to comfortably engage in activities you love.

The key is that your reason is meaningful to you. This ensures your motivation comes from a deep, intrinsic place, making it more sustainable over the long term. When the going gets tough, reminding yourself of your 'why' will reinvigorate your dedication and help you stick with your healthy habits.

Here are a few things that you can do to help yourself stay motivated and on track:

- Setting realistic goals for yourself and tracking your progress along the way is vital. Reward yourself for reaching milestones, such as losing 2 or 3 percent of your starting weight. If you have a 'bad' day, don't beat yourself up—just get back on track the next day. I read something the other day that said if you're having a bad day, it doesn't mean you are having a bad life. The same is true of diet.

- Create a plan for yourself. Write down what you plan to eat each day and make sure that you stick to your plan. This will help you make healthy choices and stay on track.

- Find a support system. This could be family, friends, or even an online community. Having people to help keep you stay motivated can be a great way to lose weight.

Bland Food — Absolutely Not!

Healthy and delicious meals don't have to be boring or complicated. The key is in using fresh, whole ingredients and adding plenty of herbs and spices for flavour. Here are just a few healthy and delicious meals ideas to get you thinking:

- **Quinoa Salad with Roasted Vegetables:** Combine a mix of cooked quinoa with your favourite roasted vegetables (like bell peppers, zucchini, and carrots), and a simple lemon vinaigrette.

- **Greek Yoghurt Chicken:** Marinate chicken breasts in Greek yogurt, lemon juice, garlic, and herbs, then bake until golden and juicy.

- **Spicy Shrimp and Avocado Lettuce Wraps:** Fill crisp lettuce leaves with spicy sautéed shrimp and avocado slices, then drizzle with a lime dressing.

- **Sweet Potato and Black Bean Tacos:** Fill soft corn tortillas with roasted sweet potato cubes, black beans, avocado, and a sprinkle of cheese.

- **Vegetable Stir Fry with Tofu:** Prepare by sauteing a medley of vegetables such as bell peppers, bok choy and peas along with tofu.

- **Baked Salmon:** Season a salmon fillet with the flavour of lemon juice, fragrant dill and a sprinkle of pepper. Bake until the salmon becomes beautifully flaky and tender.

- **Spinach and Low Sodium Feta Stuffed Chicken Breast:** Fill a chicken breast with a mixture of spinach and flavourful feta cheese. Then let it bake until fully cooked to perfection.

- **Zucchini Noodles with Pesto and Cherry Tomatoes:** Combine spiralized zucchini noodles with basil pesto, made from scratch, using fresh ingredients. Complete this light dish by adding cherry tomatoes for a burst of flavour.

- **Turkey and Quinoa Stuffed Bell Peppers:** Fill bell peppers with a mixture of ground turkey and cooked quinoa, then bake until the peppers are tender.

- **Chickpea and Vegetable Curry:** Simmer chickpeas, tomatoes, and a mix of vegetables (like cauliflower and peas) with curry spices until everything is tender and flavourful.

If you're curious, rest assured that all the recipes above align with the principles of the DASH diet. These recipes prioritise whole grains, lean proteins, vegetables, and healthy fats—all key components of a DASH-friendly meal. You can find these recipes, along with the specific ingredients and instructions, detailed in Chapter 7 of this book.

Calorie Counting — No More!

When it comes to weight loss, calorie counting is often seen as the gold standard. But is it really necessary?

The short answer is no.

There are plenty of other ways to lose weight that don't involve counting every single calorie. For example, you could simply:

- Focus on eating more nutrient-rich foods and fewer processed foods. This approach can help you automatically eat fewer calories without having to consciously think about them.

- Eat smaller portions. This doesn't mean you have to starve yourself—just be mindful of how much food you're putting on your plate.

- Engage in regular exercise—a great way to burn calories and boost your metabolism.

There you have it—weight loss doesn't have to be complicated. If you want to, just ditch the calorie counting and try one of these simpler approaches instead. We will cover more on this in the next chapter.

Keeping the Weight Off

To lose weight and **keep it off**, you need to make permanent changes to your lifestyle. Here are some things to watch out for:

- **Protein.** Make sure you are getting enough protein. Protein helps to keep you feeling full and can help to reduce cravings. Include lean protein sources such as chicken, fish, tofu, legumes, and eggs in your diet.

- **Be careful of carb creep.** Refined carbs as found in white bread, pasta, and pastries can cause blood sugar spikes and lead to cravings. Keep with the whole grain option instead. Be mindful of white foods; white bread, white rice, white pasta etc.

- **Continue to eat fruits and vegetables.** Fruits and veggies are packed with fibre, vitamins, and minerals. They are also low in calories. Include a **variety** of them in your diet for optimum health.

- **Avoid sugary drinks.** Soda, sports drinks, energy drinks, and fruit juices can contain a lot of sugar and calories. Stick to water or unsweetened tea instead.

- **Make sure you're getting enough sleep.** Lack of sleep can lead to weight gain. Aim for 7-8 hours of good quality, uninterrupted sleep, every night.

- **Avoid processed foods.** Processed foods are often high in sugar, salt, and unhealthy fats. Choose whole, unprocessed foods instead.

- **Avoid alcohol:** Alcoholic beverages can creep up on you, leading to far too many calories. An honest look at alcohol intake is required.

Consistency in maintaining eating habits and engaging in exercise will yield noticeable results within a reasonable time frame. If your goal is to lose a large amount of weight, it's important to acknowledge that achieving this within a short time period is unlikely. Instead, focus on losing a pound or two every week or month, **consistently.** Weight loss is a process that involves ups and downs along the way. Healthy weight loss takes time. **Patience is key.** It's perfectly normal to experience setbacks, or weeks where the weight doesn't seem to shift. Stay committed and persistent. Eventually, you will see results.

Planners and Trackers

Throughout this chapter, we've emphasised the importance of mindfulness in your weight loss journey. By keeping a detailed record of what you eat, and when you eat, you'll not only be able to understand your eating habits better, but also identify patterns that might be hindering your progress. To aid this process, consider using a Meal Planner and Tracker, which can make this task more organised and less daunting. Similarly, we've highlighted the significance of documenting your weight loss progress. A Weight Log and Tracker can serve as a tangible record of your hard work, reflecting the milestones you've achieved along the way. These tools can keep you motivated and focused on your goal. And here's the good news—both a Meal Planner/Tracker and Weight Log/Tracker are available for you to download, print and use, absolutely free at

https://amitylifebooks.com/dashfree

26 Weight Loss Tips

As we round this chapter off, here are some top weight loss tips for you to think about that will support your weight loss journey. Some of this may sound like repetition, but repetition is good when it comes to instilling valuable concepts, especially where habits are concerned.

1. **Eat a balanced diet:** Include a variety of fruits and vegetables. In addition, focus on lean proteins, whole grains, and healthy fats. This is the core fundamental of DASH.

2. **Portion control:** Pay attention to portion sizes to avoid overeating, even of healthy foods.

3. **Regular exercise:** Aim for at least 150 minutes of moderate aerobic activity or 75 minutes of vigorous activity each week, along with strength training exercises on two or more days a week. Breaking that down, you are looking at a 22 minute walk per day or a quick 11 minute jog around the block.

4. **Eating window control:** Try intermittent fasting, which involves limiting the hours during which you consume food. This can help reduce calorie intake and boost metabolic processes that aid in weight loss. At a minimum, concentrate on breakfast in the morning, lunch at midday and dinner in the evening.

5. **Stay hydrated:** Drinking water not only helps quench thirst but also helps manage hunger. Try fizzy water for an even fuller feeling.

6. **Avoid processed foods and sugars:** These types of foods often pack a lot of calories but lack nutrients. It's best to minimise their consumption.

7. **Prioritise quality sleep:** Getting sufficient sleep is crucial for healthy metabolism and regulating hunger hormones.

8. **Be mindful when eating:** Pay attention to what you eat and take the time to savour each bite. Avoid eating on the go, or while being distracted, as this can lead to overeating.

9. **Increase protein intake:** Including protein rich foods in your diet can help you feel fuller for longer periods and prevent excessive snacking or overeating.

10. **Regular health check-ups:** Scheduling routine medical check-ups can provide insights into your progress and allow for adjustments to be made—if necessary—to your weight loss plan.

11. **Set goals:** It's important to set achievable goals that keep you motivated along the way, helping you stay focused on long-term success, rather than quick fixes.

12. **Embrace fibre rich foods:** Incorporating fibre into your meals promotes feelings of fullness and satisfaction, aiding in appetite control throughout the day.

13. **Be cautious of 'diet' foods:** Beware of products labelled as 'low fat' or 'diet' as they may contain hidden sugars or other unhealthy additives that could hinder your weight loss efforts.

14. **Cook homemade meals whenever possible:** By preparing meals at home, you have control over the ingredients that are used. You also control the portion sizes, allowing for a healthier approach to eating.

15. **Keep a food journal:** Keeping track of what and when you eat can help identify patterns and make it easier to make the necessary adjustments.

16. **Stay consistent:** Weight loss requires time and consistent efforts. Don't get discouraged if progress seems slow; consistency is key.

17. **Spice it up:** Spices like cayenne pepper can boost metabolism and create a thermogenic effect, which can help burn calories.

18. **Eat more slowly:** It takes time for the brain to register satiety signals. Eating more slowly can help you eat less and feel fuller.

19. **Drink black coffee:** Black coffee can boost metabolism and help burn fat. Just be sure not to add sugar or cream.

20. **Use smaller plates and bowls:** This simple visual brain hack makes portions look larger, helping to curb overeating.

21. **Cutting down on alcohol:** This is advisable, as alcohol can contribute to unwanted calories. It also impairs decision making, resulting in unhealthy food choices.

22. **Consider using a standing desk:** Instead of sitting down for long periods at a desk, try standing instead. This will burn more calories and potentially aid in weight loss.

23. **Brush your teeth after meals:** Not only good for healthy teeth and gums, but this practice can also help curb the urge to snack unnecessarily.

24. **Sunlight:** Simply spending some time in the sun during the morning hours can positively impact your metabolism and mood. This can indirectly support weight loss efforts.

25. **Fermented foods**: Adding foods like yogurt, kefir or kombucha in your diet can enhance gut health. Good gut health can potentially assist with weight loss goals.

26. **Yoga or meditation:** Incorporating practices like this into your daily routine can be beneficial. Stress has been linked to weight gain through increased cortisol release (a hormone that stimulates appetite). Engaging in mindfulness activities can help manage stress levels.

Chapter Summary

As we wrap up this chapter, let's take a moment to reflect on the ground we've covered. We've delved into the science of weight loss, exploring concepts like caloric intake, sensible nutrition and demystified common misconceptions surrounding weight loss. We even explored the workings of our metabolism, learning about its impact on weight loss.

Now, you're armed with two vital things (1) fundamental knowledge and (2) understanding. These are essential tools as you navigate your weight loss journey. We've laid the groundwork and set the stage for what comes next. Talking of which, in the next chapter, we'll introduce the DASH diet. We'll explore its principles and how it can align with your weight loss goals. See you in the next chapter.

Chapter 2: Understanding the DASH Diet

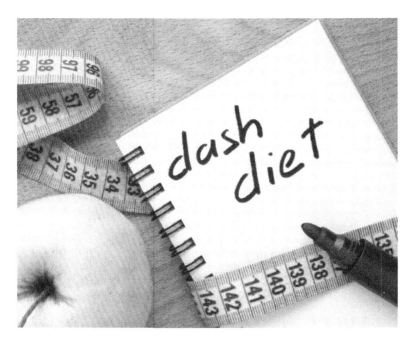

"Sorry, there's no magic bullet. You gotta eat healthy and live healthy to be healthy and look healthy. End of story."

—Morgan Spurlock[3]

As we navigate through the complexities of weight loss and health management, we encounter various dietary strategies. Some shine brightly and fade quickly, while others persist, backed by robust scientific evidence. The DASH diet, an acronym for **D**ietary **A**pproaches to **S**top **H**ypertension, distinctly belongs to the latter group.

---

[3] American documentary filmmaker and television producer (Super Size Me)

The DASH Diet Explained — Properly

The DASH diet study was initiated in 1997 by the National Heart, Lung, and Blood Institute (NHLBI). The focus was to test the effects that a diet rich in fruits, vegetables, and low-fat dairy products can have on blood pressure.

In the study, participants were divided into three groups: one following a typical American diet, another incorporating more fruits and vegetables, and a third group following the DASH diet. The results were remarkable. The study clearly showed that the DASH diet proved to be **the most effective** in reducing blood pressure. Even more promising was that reductions in blood pressure were observed within just two weeks of starting the diet. The study, entitled "A clinical trial of the effects of dietary patterns on blood pressure" concluded by stating that "a diet rich in fruits, vegetables, and low-fat dairy foods and with reduced saturated and total fat can substantially lower blood pressure" (Appel et al., 1997). This research-backed origin alone, sets the DASH diet apart from diets that often lack scientific rigour and grounding.

The primary principle behind the DASH diet is simple. Practitioners are required to consume nutrient-rich foods that provide ample amounts of potassium, calcium, and magnesium—nutrients essential in managing and lowering blood pressure. Consequently, this diet emphasises fruits, vegetables, whole grains, lean meats, and low-fat dairy products, while minimising foods high in saturated fats, trans fats, and sodium.

The nutritional profile of the DASH diet reveals a scientific approach that does not require counting calories. The DASH diet aims for a dietary pattern that includes 27% of total calories from fat (with less than 6% from saturated fat), 18% from protein, and 55% from carbohydrates. In addition, it recommends consuming less than 2,300 mg of sodium per day, eventually lowering it to 1,500 mg. It also strongly encourages exercise.

At this stage, it really should be pointed out that although the DASH diet was initially developed to lower blood pressure, you can be confident that the benefits go beyond that. Research has shown that it is effective in reducing levels of LDL cholesterol and triglycerides while improving heart health. Additionally, DASH can help lower the risk of heart disease, stroke and other cardiovascular conditions.

The efficacy of the DASH diet has been proven in numerous studies. A study published in *Obesity Reviews* concluded that the "DASH diet is a good choice for weight management particularly for weight reduction in overweight and obese participants" (Soltani et al., 2016). Another study, published in *Frontiers in Nutrition* concluded that the "DASH diet was effective in the reduction of BP and other cardiovascular risk factors, including blood glucose, blood lipids, body weight, and waist circumference" (Guo et al., 2021). Another remarkable study was published in the *Archives of Internal Medicine* which concluded that "For overweight or obese persons with above-normal BP, the addition of exercise and weight loss to the DASH diet resulted in even larger BP reductions, greater improvements in vascular and autonomic function, and reduced left ventricular mass" (Blumenthal, 2010). These are examples of studies that you can trust.

By providing a nutrient-dense, balanced eating approach that supports overall health and wellness, DASH serves as an excellent model for sustainable weight loss. Through this scientific, evidence-based lens, we'll continue to explore the potent synergistic effects of coupling the DASH diet with regular physical exercise. This is the focus of subsequent chapters.

As we delve deeper into the DASH diet, I encourage you to view it not merely as a list of "allowed" and "disallowed" foods, but as a guiding philosophy for a healthier life.

Q. But what exactly is the DASH diet and why does it work so well? Let's take a closer look.

There are two versions of the DASH diet: the standard version, and the low-sodium version. The low-sodium version (1,500 milligrams per day) is recommended for people with high blood pressure, while the standard version (2,300 milligrams per day) is meant for general healthy eating. These sodium values are limits, not targets, in case you were wondering!

Here's a guideline of portion sizes and food types that can fit into a 2,000-calorie DASH diet:

- **Grains and Grain Products:** 6-8 servings per day. An example serving could be a slice of bread, 1/2 cup of cooked rice or pasta, or 1 ounce of dry cereal.

- **Fruits:** 4-5 servings per day. An example serving might be one medium fruit, 1/2 cup fresh, frozen or canned fruit, or 4 ounces of fresh juice.

- **Vegetables:** 4-5 servings per day. An example serving could be 1 cup of raw leafy vegetables, or 1/2 cup of other vegetables (broccoli, cauliflower, etc), either cooked or raw.

- **Low-fat or Non-fat Dairy Products:** 2-3 servings per day. An example serving could be 1 cup of milk or yoghurt, or 1.5 ounces of cheese.

- **Lean Meats, Poultry, and Fish:** 6 or fewer servings per day. An example serving could be 1 ounce of cooked meats, poultry, or fish. An egg counts as one serving.

- **Nuts, Seeds, and Legumes:** 4-5 servings per week. An example serving could be 1/3 cup or 1.5 ounces of nuts, 2 tablespoons or 1/2 ounce of seeds, or 1/2 cup cooked legumes (dried beans or peas).

- **Fats and Oils:** 2-3 servings per day. An example serving could be 1 teaspoon of soft margarine, 1 tablespoon of mayonnaise, or 2 tablespoons of salad dressing.

- **Sweets and Added Sugars:** 5 or fewer servings per week. An example serving could be 1 tablespoon of sugar, 1 tablespoon of jelly or jam, or a 1/2 cup of sorbet.

Note: The National Institute of Diabetes and Digestive and Kidney Diseases (NIH) maintain serving recommendations for **other daily calorie** requirements here:

- **https://www.nhlbi.nih.gov/education/dash/follo wing-dash**

The NIH also maintains a 'Body Weight Planner' at **https://www.niddk.nih.gov/bwp** which will tell you **exactly** how many calories per day you need to consume in order to lose weight. It factors in your starting weight, height, gender and age, end goal weight, how long you want it to take, your current activity level, and your activity change level (how much exercise you plan to do). From this, it will tell you **exactly** how many calories you need to consume per day in order to reach this goal. Once you know this, it's a simple matter of heading back over to the 'DASH Eating Plan' at **https://www.nhlbi.nih.gov/education/dash/following-dash** to find the number of food servings you can eat from the food groups by calorie level. That's it! It's easy, and anyone can do this. No maths involved.

The beauty of the DASH diet lies in its simplicity and flexibility. By following the serving suggestions, there is no need to obsess over calories or exact portion sizes. Instead, the focus is on consuming a balanced variety of foods from each recommended food group. But let's be sensible here, while you don't have to meticulously count calories, consuming an excess of even healthy foods can lead to weight gain. This is why you need to follow the DASH eating plan above.

The DASH diet is about making lasting, sustainable changes to your eating habits. It's not a restrictive, quick-fix diet. Instead, it's a way of eating that supports long-term health and well-being. Following the recommended servings from each food group should naturally guide you towards a healthier pattern of eating. And as a bonus, these whole, minimally processed foods can be much more filling than their processed counterparts, which can help prevent overeating.

Stay patient, keep listening to your body's hunger and fullness cues, and remember that every step towards healthier eating is a step in the right direction!

Q. I just want to lose weight on the DASH diet. Should I be concerned with the sodium levels? Can I ignore them? I don't even have high blood pressure!

Reducing sodium in your diet doesn't directly lead to weight loss, but it does help in managing your weight **indirectly** in lots of ways:

- **Food choices:** High-sodium foods are often processed and unhealthy. Such foods contribute to weight gain. By aiming to reduce sodium, you are much more likely to lean more towards fresh fruits, vegetables, lean proteins, and whole grains. These are healthier and better for weight management. This is an undeniable fact.

- **Caloric intake:** Foods high in sodium, such as fast food and processed snacks, are also (often) high in calories and unhealthy saturated fats. Similar to avoiding sodium; by reducing your intake of such foods, you will likely decrease your overall caloric intake, again aiding in weight management.

- **Blood pressure and heart health:** A high sodium diet often leads to hypertension (high blood pressure)—a risk factor for heart disease. Heart health and weight management are closely linked. When your heart is healthy, it's much easier for you to engage in physical activity and exercise to help burn calories.

- **Water retention:** Sodium plays a crucial role in fluid balance in the body. Consuming too much sodium can cause your body to retain excess water. This can lead to bloating and a temporary increase in weight. By reducing sodium, you can decrease water retention, helping your body to maintain a more stable weight.

Even though the DASH diet is especially recommended for people with high blood pressure, it's a well-rounded approach to eating that can benefit everyone, including those trying to lose weight. While you may not have high blood pressure (yet, hopefully never), paying attention to your sodium intake is still important for overall health.

If monitoring your sodium intake feels too overwhelming whilst you are just getting started with weight loss, you could prioritise other aspects of the diet first. Your attention should be primarily be focussed on portion control, choosing whole foods, and increasing your intake of fruits, vegetables, and whole grains.

Once you feel comfortable with these changes, you can start gradually lowering your sodium intake. Small changes like removing the salt shaker from the table, reducing the amount of salt in recipes, and choosing low-sodium versions of foods will all make a significant difference.

Q. Is DASH a low carb diet?

No. The Dash diet is not a low-carb diet, but it is a lower carb diet than the typical Western diet, for example. The diet emphasises fruits, vegetables, and whole grains, which are all sources of complex carbohydrates. It does, however, include lean protein and low-fat dairy, which are excellent sources of protein and calcium, but typically contain relatively few carbs.

A Typical Day on the DASH Diet — Soon to Be Your Day

Probably the best way to understand what a DASH diet entails is to look at what an average day looks like:

- **Morning routine:** Start your day with a healthy breakfast such as whole-grain oatmeal with a side of fresh fruit.

- **Hydration:** Throughout the day, ensure you stay hydrated by drinking plenty of water. Try to avoid sugary beverages and limit caffeine intake.

- **Mindful snacking:** Prepare healthy snacks for the day. This could be fresh fruits, raw vegetables with a hummus dip, or a handful of unsalted nuts.

- **Meal planning and preparation:** Plan your lunch and dinner ahead of time. Make sure your meals are balanced, containing lean proteins, whole grains, vegetables, and a moderate amount of healthy fats. When planning meals, envision filling half your plate with colourful fruits and vegetables, a quarter with lean proteins, and the remaining quarter with whole grains. This simple visual cue can be immensely helpful in maintaining balance and variety in your diet.

- **Sodium watch:** While cooking, pay attention to the sodium content of your ingredients. Use herbs and spices for flavouring instead of salt.

- **Physical activity:** Incorporate at least 30 minutes of moderate-intensity exercise into your week day, more at the weekends if you can. This could be a brisk walk, a swim, or a bike ride.

- **Evening routine:** For dinner, prepare a meal that's rich in vegetables, whole grains, and lean proteins. Keep red meat and sugary foods to a minimum.

- **Tracking:** Before you retire for the day, write down what you have eaten in a food diary. This will help track your progress, and make necessary adjustments if required.

- **Reading labels:** Whenever you purchase food, read the labels to ensure they align with DASH guidelines (low sodium).

- **Nutrition boost:** Seek to incorporate potassium-rich foods into your meals (fruits and vegetables). We'll cover the importance of potassium later in this chapter.

Consistency is key when it comes to reaping the benefits of the DASH diet. It's not about perfect adherence every day, but about making overall healthier choices **over time.**

A Simple 7-day DASH Diet Menu Plan

To help in understanding even further, let's look in detail at a typical week. This plan gives you an idea of the types of foods you can enjoy on the DASH diet. Feel free to use this as the basis of your own 7-day plan, adjusting as required.

Day 1:

- **Breakfast:** Quinoa porridge with fresh berries and a handful of almonds.

- **Lunch:** Grilled chicken salad with mixed greens, cherry tomatoes, cucumber, and vinaigrette.

- **Dinner:** Baked salmon with lemon and dill, a side of roasted vegetables, and a serving of brown rice.

- **Snack:** Greek yoghurt with a drizzle of honey and a small apple.

Day 2:

- **Breakfast:** Whole grain toast with avocado and a boiled egg.

- **Lunch:** Turkey and quinoa stuffed bell peppers with a side of mixed greens.

- **Dinner:** Shrimp stir-fry with a variety of vegetables and a serving of brown rice.

- **Snack:** A handful of unsalted mixed nuts and a banana.

Day 3:

- **Breakfast:** Scrambled eggs with spinach and low-sodium feta (optional), served with a slice of whole grain toast.

- **Lunch:** Sweet potato and black bean tacos with a side of salsa.

- **Dinner:** Baked chicken breast with a side of quinoa salad.

- **Snack:** A cup of berries and a piece of dark chocolate.

Day 4:

- **Breakfast:** Oatmeal with almond milk, a sprinkle of cinnamon, and topped with fresh fruit.

- **Lunch:** Vegetable stir-fry with tofu served over brown rice.

- **Dinner:** Zucchini noodles with pesto and cherry tomatoes.

- **Snack:** Celery sticks with hummus and a small orange.

Day 5:

- **Breakfast:** Greek yoghurt with mixed berries and a handful of granola.

- **Lunch:** Chickpea and vegetable curry served over whole grain couscous.

- **Dinner:** Grilled fish with a side of roasted Brussels sprouts and sweet potatoes.

- **Snack:** Baby carrots and a small apple.

Day 6:

- **Breakfast:** Whole grain pancakes with a side of fresh fruit.

- **Lunch:** Grilled chicken wrap with a side of mixed greens.

- **Dinner:** Turkey meatballs with marinara sauce served over spaghetti squash.

- **Snack:** Greek yoghurt with a drizzle of honey and a banana.

Day 7:

- **Breakfast:** Egg and vegetable scramble with a slice of whole grain toast.

- **Lunch:** Greek salad with grilled chicken.

- **Dinner:** Jacket potato with a filling of your choice (no-mayo tuna and sweetcorn works well).

- **Snack:** A cup of mixed berries and a handful of unsalted almonds.

Adjust the serving sizes and add or subtract food items based on your individual calorie and nutrient needs.

Grocery Shopping List for the DASH Diet

Success with the DASH diet starts with a well-planned grocery shopping list. Your list should prioritise:

- **Fresh fruits:** Apples, Bananas, Berries (Strawberries, Blueberries, Raspberries, Blackberries), Oranges, Grapes, Pineapple, Kiwi, Mangoes, Papaya, Watermelon, Pears, Plums, Peaches, Avocados (technically a fruit), Cherries.

- **Fresh vegetables:** Spinach, Broccoli, Carrots, Sweet potatoes, Brussels sprouts, Peppers (Red, Yellow, Green), Tomatoes, Cucumbers, Zucchini, Squash, Kale, Beets, Eggplant, Cauliflower, Lettuce (Romaine, Butterhead, Iceberg), Arugula, Asparagus, Green beans.

- **Whole grains:** Choose brown rice, whole-wheat pasta, and whole grain bread or cereals. Other grains include Quinoa, Whole oats/oatmeal, Whole grain barley, Whole grain rye, Freekeh, Buckwheat, Bulgur (cracked wheat), Millet, Sorghum, Whole wheat pasta, Whole grain bread, Wild rice, Spelt, Teff, Amaranth, Farro, Whole grain cornmeal, Kamut.

- **Lean proteins:** This includes poultry, fish, and lean cuts of meat such as Chicken breast, Turkey breast, Fish (such as salmon, tuna, and cod), Shellfish (like shrimp and lobster), Lean cuts of beef (such as eye of round, top round, bottom round, and sirloin), Lean cuts of pork (like pork loin or tenderloin), Eggs (particularly egg whites), Low-fat dairy products (such as milk, yoghurt, and cottage cheese), Tofu, Legumes (like lentils, chickpeas, and black beans), Quinoa, Edamame, Seitan, Tempeh, Greek yoghurt, Venison, Bison, Skinless Turkey, Skinless Chicken Thigh, Low-fat Cottage Cheese, Protein powder (whey, casein, or plant-based).

- **Low-fat or non-fat dairy:** These foods provide you with necessary calcium and vitamin D.

- **Nuts, seeds, and legumes:** These are excellent sources of protein and fibre.

- **Healthy fats and oils:** Avocado, Olive, Canola (Rapeseed), Flaxseed, Walnut, Chia Seed, Almond, Sesame, Sunflower, Hemp.

Reading Food Labels and Avoiding Hidden Sodium

High sodium intake can lead to elevated blood pressure and therefore reading food labels becomes an important factor in following this guideline. When reading a food label, look at the 'Nutrition Facts' panel. Pay close attention to the 'Sodium' line, listed in milligrams (mg) and the '% Daily Value'. The % Daily Values will be based on a 2,000 calorie diet in case you were wondering. To make sure you stay within the guideline, choose products with a sodium Daily Value of 5% or less. Obviously, your daily values may be higher or lower depending on your calorie needs, but this is a good rule of thumb. Let's keep it simple!

As an exercise, look at the nutritional value for this example canned food item below:

Nutrition Facts

Serving Size: 1 cup (240g)

Servings Per Container: About 2

Amount Per Serving:

- Calories: 150

- Total Fat: 3 g (4% Daily Value)

- Saturated Fat: 1 g (5% Daily Value)

- Trans Fat: 0 g

- Cholesterol: 20 mg (7% Daily Value)

- Sodium: 900 mg **(**39% Daily Value**)**

- Total Carbohydrate: 22 g (8% Daily Value)

- Dietary Fibre: 3 g (11% Daily Value)

- Sugars: 4 g

- Includes Added Sugars: 2g (4% Daily Value)

- Protein: 8 g

- Vitamin D: 0 mcg (0% Daily Value)

- Calcium: 60 mg (5% Daily Value)

- Iron: 1.2 mg (7% Daily Value)

- Potassium: 300 mg (6% Daily Value)

This product has a high sodium content, clocking in at 900 mg per serving. This accounts for a substantial 39% of the recommended daily intake of sodium based on the 2,300 mg limit. At the same time, the potassium level is relatively low at just 300 mg per serving, which only fulfils around 6% of the recommended daily value. **Potassium plays an essential role** in maintaining healthy blood pressure levels, as it helps to counteract the blood pressure-raising effects of sodium. A diet rich in potassium can potentially help to lower blood pressure and reduce the risk of heart disease. The high sodium to low potassium ratio in this product certainly isn't optimal for someone who is conscious about their sodium intake and concerned about blood pressure.

Please note that nutritional values will vary significantly based on the specific product, so it's always important to read the label on the specific product you are consuming. To be clear, not all products are created equal.

Sodium can be sneaky! Foods like bread, canned soups, and cold cuts often contain more sodium than you might expect. Beware of terms like 'soda' (as in baking soda, it means sodium bicarbonate), 'monosodium glutamate', 'sodium nitrate', 'sodium citrate', 'sodium benzoate' as these are all sources of dietary sodium.

The DASH diet is about more than just individual nutrients; it's about a healthier pattern of eating. Prepare for it thoughtfully, shop for groceries mindfully, and be aware of hidden sodium. With these strategies, you'll be well on your way to embracing the DASH lifestyle and all the health benefits it brings.

Enjoying Desserts on the DASH Diet Without Feeling Guilty

Who says a healthy diet doesn't leave room for dessert? Not the DASH diet! In fact, there are a number of sweet treats you can enjoy. I've rounded up seven of my favourite dessert recipes that align with the principles of the DASH diet. They offer a good blend of taste and nutrition.

- **Baked Apples with Cinnamon:** A simple yet satisfying dessert, baked apples are naturally sweet and packed with fibre. Core four medium-sized apples and place them in a baking dish. Sprinkle them with a mix of 1 teaspoon of cinnamon and 1-2 tablespoons of honey. Bake for 30 minutes at 350°F, or until the apples are tender.

- **Dark Chocolate Covered Strawberries:** Dark chocolate is rich in antioxidants and strawberries are packed with vitamins. Melt 1 bar (about 100 grams) of dark chocolate (70% or higher cacao) and dip 20 strawberries, placing them on a baking sheet lined with parchment paper. Refrigerate until the chocolate has set. Get in quick before they all get eaten!

- **Greek Yoghurt Parfait:** Layer 1 cup of non-fat Greek yoghurt, 1 cup of mixed berries (fresh or frozen), and 2 tablespoons of honey in a serving glass. Top with 2 tablespoons of chopped nuts (walnuts or pecans work well) for added crunch and a dose of healthy fats.

- **Banana and Almond Butter Ice Cream:** For a cool treat, blend 2 frozen bananas and 2 tablespoons of almond butter until smooth. Freeze the mixture for 2 hours, and enjoy a dessert that's naturally sweet, high in potassium, and contains healthy fats.

- **Homemade Fruit Salad:** Mix a variety of your favourite fruits (3 cups' worth). Think berries, orange segments, apple slices, and grapes. Drizzle with 1 tablespoon of honey and the juice of one lime. Refrigerate for 1 hour before serving.

- **Chia Seed Pudding:** Combine a 1/4 cup of chia seeds with 1 cup of almond milk and 1 tablespoon of honey. Let the mixture sit in your fridge overnight. In the morning, you'll have a fibre-rich pudding that can be topped with fresh fruit.

- **Whole Grain Banana Muffins:** In a bowl, mash 3 ripe bananas and mix with a 1/3 cup of unsweetened applesauce, 2 cups of whole wheat flour, 1/2 cup of honey and 1 teaspoon of baking soda. Scoop the batter into muffin tins and bake at 350°F for around 20 minutes.

While these desserts are healthier options, portion control is key!

Chapter Summary

Congratulations! You've successfully navigated through everything you need to know to get started on the DASH Diet.

Hopefully, by now you have read enough to realise that DASH is not just a tool for hypertension control, but also a viable and scientifically-supported strategy for weight loss. Your journey with DASH isn't just about the number on the scale, but about long-term health benefits and creating sustainable, healthy habits. DASH is easy to follow and can be adapted to individual needs. You can still enjoy your favourite foods; you just need to be mindful of portion sizes.

Now that you're equipped with this wealth of knowledge, you're ready to combine the DASH diet and the healthy lifestyle it represents with physical activity. Onward to the next chapter!

Chapter 3: Exercise for Weight Loss

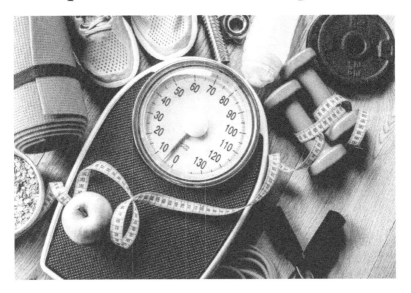

"Exercise is a journey, not a destination. It must be continued for the rest of your life. We do not stop exercising because we grow old—we grow old because we stop exercising."

—Kenneth H. Cooper[4]

So, exercise and a healthy diet are two peas in a pod I like to call *"The Blueprint for Weight Loss"*. While you will be able to shed some extra weight by opting for either option, the results you will enjoy are so much more rewarding when you combine the two.

The question that remains on the lips of many is, "How much exercise is necessary to support my weight-loss effort?" Some

---

[4] Medical doctor, renowned for his groundbreaking research on the health benefits and improvements gained from regular aerobic exercise

people have the idea that only sweating away in a gym for hours constitutes exercise. This scenario may not necessarily be the truth, as it is not *your truth*.

If you have not been exercising at all, the idea of going to a gym may be so agonising that you simply do nothing at all. If you identify as the kind of person I am describing here, it is important to realise that just getting off the couch and going for a brisk walk around the block, or in a nearby park, will also constitute exercise!

As we delve into the role of exercise in weight loss and overall health, it's essential to recognise the profound interconnection between physical activity and human physiology. Exercise isn't merely a tool to burn calories, but a catalyst that propels us toward better health and longevity.

In this chapter, I want to dissect exercise and physical activity and explore it in detail. The aim is to provide you with all the detail you need to understand it, and get going with it. We are going to cover the health benefits you can obtain from regular exercise. We will learn about exercise and weight loss, and how one helps the other. We will also cover different types of exercise; and safety tips for when you are ready to start. In fact, we are going to condense an entire book into one chapter, so get ready!

Don't stint on this chapter! Whilst you read, think how you can incorporate one or more of these activities into your daily routine. Each small change will make a big impact on your health and well-being.

The Health Benefits of Exercise — Sweat Today, Smile Tomorrow

Picture this: you're on a road trip to Better Health, with Weight Loss as your destination. Now, a nutrient-dense, balanced diet like the DASH diet might be your vehicle of choice—but exercise? Well, that's the turbo charged engine that gets you there faster, smoother, and with more benefits than you initially signed up for.

Exercise is truly a gold pot when it comes to the health benefits you can enjoy. What makes it even better is that you don't have to wait weeks before enjoying the benefits that are up for grabs. In fact, the health benefits of being active kick in immediately after your first physical activity. Let's talk about some of the benefits you will see along the way:

Improved Mental and Emotional State

When you are active and you get your heart rate to speed up, your body releases a bunch of feel-good hormones in your brain. These hormones reduce your stress levels and increase your sense of joy, contentment, and excitement about life. You may also experience an increase in your confidence to achieve the goals you have set out to accomplish. I am, of course, referring to hormones like serotonin, dopamine and endorphins. Perhaps you are familiar with the term "runner's high." These are the hormones causing this elevation in your emotions.

According to the Centers for Disease Control and Prevention (CDC, n.d.-a), being physically active also improves mental clarity and clearer thinking, and it reduces anxiety and the symptoms of depression.

The benefit you should never underestimate is the feeling of mental and emotional wellness. This is enough to give you a second and far healthier take on life.

Minimised Odds of Health Risks

There are several potentially severe health risks you may be able to avoid simply by being more active. Most of these concerns, unfortunately, rank high on the list of the deadliest diseases.

Cardiovascular disease mostly refers to either heart attacks or strokes. Both diseases—often resulting in disability or death—can be greatly reduced by making exercise a habit in your life. By being active, you reduce your 'bad' cholesterol level and lower your blood pressure; both playing a role in determining the state of your cardiovascular health. It's not enough to just say "exercise more". Let's be specific, shall we? To enjoy these benefits, you need to be active **for at least** 150 minutes per week. This is not a great deal of time, as this only equates to 30 minutes of exercise, 5 days a week (CDC, n.d.-a). It's a great reward for a minimum of investment.

Preventing Various Cancers

Even though we have seen the most astounding advances in the field of modern medicine, there are still many cancers without any cure, and even when there are cures available, the treatment is harsh and not always completely effective. When it comes to cancer in any form, prevention remains a better route than seeking a cure.

Regular physical activity is a form of prevention, which may inhibit cancers like bladder, breast, kidney, lung, colon, stomach, oesophagus, and endometrial (the lining of the uterus) cancers. If you have already won the battle with cancer and are in remission, increasing your level of physical activity **may** also help you to prevent cancer from reoccurring.

In a comprehensive study published in the Journal of the *American Medical Association*, physical activity was associated with a lower risk of 13 types of cancer. In their conclusion, they stated that "These findings support promoting physical activity as a key component of population-wide cancer prevention and control efforts." (Moore et al., 2016). If that's not a reason to put on your running shoes, what is?

Metabolic Syndrome and Type 2 Diabetes

Metabolic syndrome is linked to a wider waistline due to an accumulation of fat in the belly area. There are risks of this kind of fat, risks like high blood pressure, cholesterol concerns, and high blood sugar, with the latter being linked to type 2 diabetes. By being active for only 150 minutes a week, you can reduce the chances of either concern substantially (CDC, n.d.-a).

Better Future Health

'Bone density' and 'muscle loss' are two terms which gain importance as we age. Due to the normal physical ageing process, we gradually lose bone density, and lose muscle mass. The cause of this? Well, as we age, our bodies undergo various hormonal changes. For instance, in women, the decrease in oestrogen levels after the menopause can accelerate bone loss, potentially leading to conditions like osteoporosis. In both men and women, the age-related decline in growth hormones and testosterone levels can contribute to muscle loss, a condition known as sarcopenia. The process of ageing is sadly associated with lower levels of physical activity; further leading to the loss of bone density and muscle mass.

Fortunately, these concerns can be addressed through regular weight-bearing and resistance exercises, adequate protein intake, and ensuring sufficient intake of key nutrients like calcium and vitamin D. This is sounding very similar to the DASH diet!

Exercise Improves Mobility and Balance

As we grow older, our body may become stiff due to deterioration in the joints. The 'solution' for many people in this situation is to minimise movement due to the discomfort. This is also known as 'doing very little'. This strategy will only worsen the condition. Movement is key; the more you move, the longer you will remain mobile. Not only are you toning your muscles when you move your body, you are also improving your balance and minimising the chances of having a fall—a serious concern in later life.

Exercise Reduces the Concerns Linked to Disease

There are a range of symptoms linked to health concerns that will improve once you become more active. These concerns include pain, blood pressure, and sugar levels; and exercise can even improve nerve damage (CDC, n.d.-a).

Brain Health

I am continually astounded by the powerful impact exercise has on brain health.

Exercise prompts an array of physiological changes that have a direct and beneficial effect on our brains. It boosts blood flow, delivering more oxygen and nutrients to our brain cells. This is vital for optimal functioning. Moreover, exercise spurs on the creation of new neurons, particularly in the hippocampus, a region of the brain associated with learning and memory. This process, known as neurogenesis, can enhance cognitive abilities and protect against cognitive decline as we age. (Mandolesi et al., 2018).

Exercise and Weight Loss — Where Fat Takes an Exit

Exercise and weight loss, of course, is at the core of this book. Exercise helps to increase the rate of weight loss in two ways. As we covered in chapter 1; when you want to lose weight, you have to reduce your calorie intake to the point where you are consuming fewer calories than your body needs to sustain itself. Once your body depletes its supply of calories on hand, it turns to fat resources to use as fuel. By adding exercise to your daily routine, you increase the number of calories your body needs to sustain itself. But as you are on a calorie-conscious eating plan—this can be 2,000 calories per day like our example guideline—or less, your body will need extra energy, and faster! This all combines to burn off fat much quicker.

Now, a word of caution. Don't be disheartened **if** your weight rises for a period of time while you are engaged in a fitness regimen. This is mostly due to an increase in water weight gain brought on by exercise. It's a well-documented and common phenomenon. Instead, focus on the change in body composition, noticeable through how your clothes fit, or your progress in strength and endurance. It's a clear example of why the scale doesn't always reflect the full story of what's happening within your body. If you look good and feel good, which I am sure you will, weight loss and readjustment is working as planned!

Different Types of Exercise

There are many forms of exercise, and we can divide them mostly into the following five types:

- Aerobic training

- Strength training

- Balance and stability training

- Coordination and agility training

- Flexibility and mobility training

Aerobic Training

This kind of exercise aims to increase your heart rate and expand your lung capacity. Typically, you will do aerobic training in short bouts of exercise of one minute at a time or less. It is called "aerobic exercise," as your body relies on the oxygen you inhale for energy creation. This type of exercise is bound to make you sweat (this is perfectly normal), get your heart rate up, and make you feel great. Aerobic exercise can be a lot of work, but if you are new to it, you can start small. Start with shorter sessions and have fun! There are many fun types of activities that fall under this category: You can try cycling, dancing, rowing, hiking, jogging, swimming, or joining an aerobics class. If aerobic exercises are your thing, a beneficial benchmark to aim for is that magic 150 minutes each week. This will give you the best start on your weight-loss journey.

Strength Training

The primary purpose of this kind of exercise is to increase muscle mass. It will transform your body to be leaner, stronger, and more flexible. It will also sharpen your mind and lift your spirits. This specific category can also be divided into more subdivisions:

- **Weight-bearing exercise:** This demands that you use your body weight to push away from gravity to increase your muscle strength. While doing so, you will work on specific body parts to increase your strength and agility. Typical examples of this form of exercise are climbing stairs, hiking, and rope jumping, but also squats and even some yoga poses.

- **Non-weight-bearing exercise:** This refers to exercise where you will be sitting or even lying down. The biggest benefit is that this form of activity reduces the impact on your joints. If you are struggling with joint pain, this may be the perfect solution for you—rowing, leg presses, bicep curls, and hamstring curls are examples. For this specific form of exercise, you may need access to gym equipment. If you're not familiar with these terms, a gym induction will quickly bring you up to speed.

- **Callisthenics:** Callisthenics is a form of resistance training that leverages your own body weight to build muscle mass, strength, flexibility, and physical endurance. This discipline involves performing a variety of movements, such as pushing, pulling, jumping, or swinging, with minimal equipment, making it highly adaptable and accessible. Routine activities in callisthenics might include push-ups, pull-ups, squats, lunges, and jumping jacks. This form of exercise can make it very easy to get a great workout at home, as you do not have to rely on gym equipment.

- **Weightlifting:** This is, of course, in a class of its own. The number of exercises you can do with weights are vast and all of them burn calories, increasing both muscle mass and bone density. When you start with weightlifting, it is best to start with lighter weights and do more repetitions to give your muscles time to get stronger—this way, you will also prevent injury. Some examples are dumbbell lunges, bench presses, deadlifts, and kettlebell swings. Again, a gym induction will cover all this. If they don't, just ask.

Balance and Stability Training

Exercises falling into this category improve muscle strength and balance, and therefore you will be burning fat faster. It is easy to do these exercises without any equipment, but often it may be best to start with a qualified trainer to be sure you have your posture correct. Due to the nature of these exercises, you can perform some of them at the office or at home while working; for example, sitting on a stability ball. Other exercises include certain yoga poses and tai chi.

Coordination and Agility Training

These exercises are aimed at improving reflexes and to help prevent falls, which, as mentioned previously, are especially important to avoid in later life. Coordination and agility training can also be combined with rapid movement that will help to burn calories and lead to an increase in muscle mass. Try side steps, lateral crossovers, or quick feet as fun ways to get fit:

- **Side Steps:** Start by standing straight with your feet hip-width apart. Keep your back straight and step out to one side with one foot and then bring your other foot to join it, moving sideways. Go left or right for a few steps or more, then back again. You can increase the intensity of this exercise by picking up the pace. Resistance bands have become a popular addition to this exercise, and in fact, to agility training in general.

- **Lateral Crossovers:** Start by standing with your feet shoulder-width apart. Keeping your upper body straight, step to the side with one foot. Then, cross the other foot behind the leading foot. After this, step out with your leading foot again and bring the back foot to its original position. You can perform these steps at a jogging pace for more cardio benefit. Lateral crossovers are often performed on a step for increased difficulty.

- **Quick Feet:** Also known as fast feet, you start by standing with your feet hip-width apart and knees slightly bent. Then, quickly run in place while emphasising the speed and turnover of your feet. Your feet should be hitting the ground as quickly as possible, and it should feel like you are 'fluttering' above the ground. This is also a fantastic warm-up routine.

Flexibility and Mobility Training

These exercises increase the level of muscle and joint **movement** you have. It consists of stretching and toning of muscles and exercising (or moving) joints to allow them to move through their full range of motion.

If this is your first time learning about all these different forms of exercise, you may be feeling light-headed just reading about them! However, I felt it was important to share this relatively comprehensive presentation. Hopefully, whilst reading, you were able to pick something out that sounded like a good fit.

Being physically active doesn't mean you have to belong to a gym or need to be an outdoors person. There is literally a form of exercise for every person to choose from and an n exercise that considers all fitness levels, states of health, and caters for those with disabilities.

Q. Does increasing your activity level always entail that you have to do *formal* exercise?

No! You can also choose to increase your activity by being creative. Dancing classes are one such example. If you prefer, choose gardening as a way to get fit until you are ready to try other forms of exercise. Mowing the lawn, pruning, digging and cutting logs can be seriously labour intensive! And lets not forget sports.

Moderate Exercise Compared to Vigorous

These are the two most common ways in which exercise level is defined. *Moderate exercise* refers to any form of exercise that increases your heart rate, but not so much that you cannot talk anymore. Again, depending on your fitness level, this can be taking a brisk walk, working in your garden, a short cycle ride on the flat, or just tidying up around the house. *Vigorous exercise* is more demanding and it increases your heart rate and breathing to the point where you can no longer have a conversation. For this, we are talking about running, rope jumping, and cycling uphill. All this may sound silly, but this is the best way to know if you've moved from moderate to vigorous exercise. If you got out of breath today, then pat yourself on the back. If you can't remember when you last got out of breath, well, there is always today.

Tips Regarding Safety and Sustainability

Embarking on a weight loss journey, which includes exercise, is an exciting venture, but it's imperative to keep your health and safety in the foreground of all your activities. This section contains essential tips designed to safeguard your well-being and promote sustainable practices. Sometimes, it may take a couple of days, or even weeks to get yourself mentally prepared to start your exercise regime, so the worst thing to happen once you do is to cause yourself an injury. Injuries can vary in severity, with some likely to put you on the couch for a while. It is better, therefore, to take the following precautionary measures to heart when you decide to get active. Whether you're new to the fitness world or a seasoned pro, these insights will serve as valuable reminders to keep you on track towards achieving your health goals.

- Discuss your plans with your doctor. If you are diagnosed with a medical concern or age is not on your side, this should be a priority. Your personal doctor will be able to guide you on what you can realistically do, and what forms of exercise are best to avoid. Plans to run the local marathon should definitely be discussed!

- Never just jump into a routine (no pun intended). A safe way to start is to set at least 10 minutes apart to warm up your muscles. When muscles are cold, you are at a far greater risk of suffering from an injury. Allowing the same amount of time to cool down is just as important, and it will reduce the amount of stiffness and muscle aches you experience the next day. Even if you are only taking a brisk walk, start with a stroll and gradually up your pace and wind down in the same manner when you are nearing the end.

- Even if you have been exercising for a while, but—due to any number of reasons—have fallen out of your routine, start at a slower pace than where you left off. I've experienced this myself. I used to be able to walk 20 miles in one session. After a break of some time, I was disheartened to find that 10 miles was more than enough. Fitness quickly comes back though.

- Become more mindful and listen to your body. It is always good to push yourself a little beyond the point where it is still comfortable, but not to overdo it. If you need to take a rest day, do so. This will benefit you far more than just pushing through.

- Make sure to wear clothes that are comfortable that will not restrain your movement. Wear shoes that are suited for the exercise you are planning to do to prevent unnecessary strain or injury.

- Hydrate your body enough. If you know you are going to be sweating, take enough water along. Your body will be losing a lot of liquid by sweating and you need to replenish this to avoid dehydration. **Caution:** electrolytes contain high levels of sodium.

These tips will make exercising a safe venture, but how can you ensure that it becomes a sustainable habit?

Yes, for sure, you will be motivated the first couple of times, but it is only normal to feel a lack of this initial enthusiasm after a while. When I know that a task will demand a lot of me and take me completely out of my comfort zone, I like to list a couple of reasons why I am committing to the task. I place this list of reasons where I can see it. The fridge door works well. It's good to remind ourselves of our 'why' for inspiration. The following tips will help make things more sustainable for you:

- Select routines and exercises that are fun. There are so many different ways you can increase your level of activity, and it always helps if it's something you have an interest in and complements your personality. If you like to have someone telling you what to do, hire a fitness trainer; if you like to spend time in nature, go for a walk, or jog in the park; and if you like to be more creative and get fit without strict rules, then go dancing. It doesn't matter what you do, as long as you burn the extra calories and increase those feel-good hormones.

- Find a partner to exercise with you. Having an exercise buddy can be fun, but can also be the encouragement you need on the days when you really just don't feel like getting active. By having someone exercise with you, you are likely to remain more committed.

- Pick a convenient solution that works best for you. Whatever you decide to do, be sure that you do not have to travel far to do it, that it is convenient to fit in, and preferably is located on your daily route. The same goes for money: If you have to invest a lot of money in getting the right gear before you can start, this may become an unnecessary delay (or an excuse).

- Treat exercise like any other important appointment. Schedule your workouts in advance, and stick to them.

- Track your progress in a journal. As we've covered, the scale may not always be the most accurate reflection of your progress. It helps to also keep a record of your activity—what you have actually done. If you could only complete a 20-minute brisk walk when you started out, but are now quite comfortable maintaining the same speed for 40 minutes, this is progress you can celebrate.

Try to keep an estimated track of the calories you have burned after your workout. There are several apps will help you in this regard, but just for reference's sake, the following indicates the average amount of calories someone would burn during 30 minutes of the following exercises (CDC, n.d.-b):

- Brisk walking: 140

- Hiking: 185

- Dancing: 165

- Jogging: 295

- Aerobics: 240

- Cycling: 295

- Swimming: 255

Measuring Your Heart Rate

One way to know that you are actually burning calories while working out is to track your heart rate. By pushing your heart rate to a certain level, you can be sure that you've had a successful workout session. To enjoy optimal calorie burning, the following will give you an estimate of where you need to get your heart rate to:

- What is your age in years?

- Subtract the number from 220.

- Then take 60 and 80% of that number as an indication of what your heart rate should be.

As a hypothetical example, let's say you are 40 years old. When you subtract that from 220, you will be left with 180. Divide 180 by 10 to give you 18. Then multiply 18 by 6 and then do the same, this time by 8. This will give you your optimal heart rate window. In this case, it would be between 108 and 144 (Kerr, 2012). By ensuring an activity level that brings your heart rate to your optimal level, you can also be sure that you are burning the maximum number of calories for the activity of your choice.

Five Exercise and Weight-Loss Myths

When it comes to using exercise as a way to shed extra weight, you are bound to come across several myths, probably from well-meaning friends. While these can come across as rather innocent, they do hold the power to throw you off your tracks. So, let's bust them straight away.

Myth #1: Intense daily training brings faster results

There is a widespread belief based on the idea that if a little of something is good, then a lot of it must be great. From this mindset, the myth was born that intense exercise day after day will bring about even faster weight loss. This myth implies that your exercise regime should include no off days. While it is false, it can also be harmful to exercise in this way daily. First of all, having no off days will quickly become overwhelming and increase the odds that at some point you will feel you just had enough and cannot sustain the routine any longer. Furthermore, your body needs days to rest and recover. After every workout, your body must repair its muscles, and this can take up to 72 hours (Malacoff, 2021).

This advice should not be construed as an excuse for simply doing nothing on your rest days, or announcing that you won't be walking the dog! Let's be sensible here. If you are really hammering it at the gym, you are going to require rest, but if you are just doing low to moderate exercise, then there is no harm in making this part of your regular daily routine.

Myth #2: Crunches are the best approach to reduce your waistline

If your body tends to carry fat around your waistline, you have what is known as the typical apple body shape. A common goal for people with this shape is the desire to reduce the size of the waist. If you are exposed to the myth that the solution you seek is provided by doing as many crunches as possible, then you are likely going to believe just that, but your efforts will be in vain. First, you now know that the best way to address the risky fat collection around your waistline is through healthy eating. Added to that, you can do crunches to strengthen your core, but your core (or six-pack) consists of more than one muscle group! They all need exercise to develop the waistline and the strong core you desire.

Myth #3—The core purpose of exercise is weight loss

While it is evident that you can enhance your weight-loss efforts by adding exercise to your routine to speed up the results of your weight loss, weight loss is not the primary, or only purpose of exercise. The reason I want to bust this myth is because I believe it places you in the risky position of giving up on exercise or slipping more often in your routine. The outcome of this will likely be that you will start to gain weight again, but you will also rob yourself of many other benefits. I am specifically referring here to benefits like improved overall health—mentally and physically—feeling stronger, having better balance, being more confident, and the list continues. Exercise is a way to have a positive body image and experience, a practice that can truly enhance your quality of life, whether you have extra weight to lose, or not.

Myth #4—Stopping exercise turns muscle into fat

For as long as you are exercising, especially when doing strength-building exercises, you will gain muscle mass and lose fat. The muscles you are building are not replacing or transforming the fat tissue in your body. Fat is literally burned into fuel while muscle mass increases due to the exercise. So, when you stop exercising, the muscle will get floppy and shrink but does not turn into fat tissue. Fat tissue may also start to accumulate as you are probably consuming more calories than your body needs now you are less active, but never ever does muscle turn into fat.

Myth #5—You have to exercise long enough to see results

This myth is based on almost a similar belief as myth #1—that quantity is better than quality. Yet, it is not the case, and if you are going to allow this belief to determine your level of activity, you may very well never be able to get active. Yes, for sure, being active for a longer session will be beneficial, but it is not the only way you are going to lose weight. If you only have 30 minutes a day, take those 30 minutes and make the most of them. I even want to say that if the only time you have is to rather take the stairs than get into the lift, or go on a lunchtime walk, then do just that. Every activity you partake in burns more calories and will help you to reach your target weight.

Suitable Exercises for Different Fitness Levels

While it's critical to find exercises that you genuinely enjoy, it's equally important to choose ones that are safe and effective based on where you currently stand on the fitness scale. So, let's get down to science and explore suitable exercises for different fitness levels.

Beginners

Low-impact workouts are a gentle, effective way to begin, providing a good foundation for cardiovascular health and muscular strength without overly stressing the joints.

- **Walking:** One of the most recommended exercises for beginners is walking. It's low-impact, requires no special equipment, and can be done anywhere. Start with a 5-10 minute walk and gradually build up to 30 minutes a day.

- **Swimming:** Water-based activities, like swimming or water aerobics, are also great options. These activities are gentle on the joints while still providing resistance to work your muscles.

- **Yoga:** Yoga is another beginner-friendly exercise. It's excellent for improving balance, flexibility, and mindfulness.

- **Lightweight Strength Training:** The use of light weights or resistance bands targeting the major muscle groups is a great form of beginner exercise—aim for 2-3 sessions per week.

Low-intensity exercise can lead to significant health improvements if done **consistently**.

Intermediate

Intermediate forms of exercise incorporate a level of difficulty beyond beginner level workouts, but are not as intense or complex as advanced routines. Here are some examples for when you have built up a basic fitness level.

- **Cycling:** Whether outdoor or stationary, cycling can help improve cardiovascular health, leg strength and joint mobility.

- **Jogging:** This is a moderate-intensity cardiovascular exercise that is a step-up from walking.

- **Bodyweight Exercises:** Push-ups, squats, lunges, and planks with variations.

- **Yoga/Pilates:** Intermediate classes will incorporate more challenging poses and sequences.

- **Strength Training with Weights:** Lifting heavier weights or implementing more complex moves like overhead presses, deadlifts, or squats.

Advanced

If you're an advanced exerciser, it means you have a high level of fitness and can therefore handle more intense and complex movements such as:

- **HIIT:** High-intensity interval training (HIIT) involves short, intense bursts of exercise followed by brief recovery periods. This type of training can lead to **significant** improvements in aerobic fitness, muscular strength, and body composition.

- **Circuit Training:** A combination of intense strength and cardio exercises performed in sequence with little to no rest in between. Classes are widely available.

- **Jumping Rope:** Don't be fooled by the name; this is a high-intensity workout that improves cardiovascular health, agility, and coordination.

- **Boxing or Kickboxing Training:** These are intense full-body workouts that improve strength, speed, agility, and cardiovascular health and no, you don't need to fight anyone!

- **Other:** Advanced activities including endurance running, power yoga, and other more advanced forms of weightlifting.

If you are already well into a fitness regime, try to include a mix of cardio, strength training, and flexibility exercises into your regime for all-round and balanced fitness.

Designing and Creating an Exercise Plan

Physical activity is an integral part of any health journey, and when combined with the DASH diet, it can yield phenomenal results. Research indicates that people who have **specific exercise schedules** are more likely to stick to their routines. A well-designed exercise plan provides the structure to ensure that you're engaging in a balanced approach to physical fitness. The exact plan for you requires a thoughtful understanding of your current fitness level, health status, and personal goals.

Here is an example 7-day exercise routine designed for **intermediate to advanced** level individuals focusing on weight loss:

Day 1: Strength Training

- **Warm-Up:** 10-minute brisk walking or jogging

- **Workout:** 30 minutes of full-body strength training (push-ups, pull-ups, lunges, squats, deadlifts, bench press)

- **Cool Down:** 10 minutes of stretching

Day 2: Cardio and Core

- **Warm-Up:** 10 minutes light jogging

- **Workout:** 30 minutes of high-intensity interval training (HIIT) cardio, 15 minutes core workout (planks, crunches, Jumping Jacks)

- **Cool Down:** 10 minutes of stretching

Day 3: Active Recovery

- 30-45 minutes of light activity, such as walking, yoga, or tai chi

Day 4: Strength Training

- **Warm-Up:** 10-minute brisk walking or jogging

- **Workout:** 30 minutes of full-body strength training (push-ups, pull-ups, lunges, squats, deadlifts, bench press)

- **Cool Down:** 10 minutes of stretching

Day 5: Cardio and Core

- **Warm-Up:** 10 minutes light jogging

- **Workout:** 30 minutes of high-intensity interval training (HIIT) cardio, 15 minutes core workout (planks, bicycle crunches, Jumping Jacks)

- **Cool Down:** 10 minutes of stretching

Day 6: Pilates or Yoga (Rest Day)

- 60-minute Pilates or yoga class focusing on strength and flexibility

Day 7: Active Recovery (Rest Day)

- 30-45 minutes of light activity, such as walking, yoga, or tai chi

Creating an exercise plan isn't about crafting it perfectly on the first attempt; it's about ongoing learning, adjusting, and finding what works best for you. Adjust the plan as needed based on how your body feels and responds. This is your plan. Stay safe, have fun, and embrace the journey towards a healthier you!

To help you record the exercise you actually do, there is a Weekly Exercise Planner and Log ready for you to print out and use. Download it for free at:

https://amitylifebooks.com/dashfree

Exercising at Home — The Kitchen Cardio

Exercising at home is convenient, cost-effective, and private. You don't have to worry about what you think you look like, or how you think you are performing in front of other people. These weight loss exercises are ideal do at home:

Leg Swings

Leg swings are a great warm-up exercise to activate your hip muscles and increase your range of motion.

Start by standing next to a wall or any sturdy support that you can hold on to for balance. Stand tall and maintain a slight bend in your supporting leg. Swing the other leg forward and backward in a smooth, controlled motion. Try to swing your leg as high as it can comfortably go, but not forcefully, or let the motion control your movement. Allow your hips to open up with each swing. Perform about 10-15 swings, then switch to the other leg.

You can also do side-to-side leg swings. For this, face the wall or support, and swing your leg across your body, and then out to the side. Again, the goal is not to swing your leg as high or as fast as possible, but simply to warm up your hip joint and muscles.

Jumping Jacks

This is a classic cardio exercise that gets your heart rate up in no time. All you need is a little bit of space to do them.

Start by standing with your feet together and your arms at your sides. Then, jump up and spread your legs out wide while bringing your arms up over your head. You can clap your hands together if you like. Jump back to the starting position and repeat.

Squats

Squats are a great strength-training exercise for your lower body. They work your quads, hamstrings, and glutes. They can also help improve your balance and coordination.

Start by standing with your feet shoulder-width apart and your arms at your sides. Then, lower your backside down towards the ground like you're going to sit in a chair. Once your thighs are parallel to the ground, push back up to the starting position.

Push-ups

Push-ups work your entire upper body, including your chest, shoulders, arms, and core. They're also a great way to improve your posture.

Start in a plank position, facing the floor, with your hands shoulder-width apart and your feet hip-width apart. Lower your chest down towards the ground. Keep your core engaged, and your back straight. Once your chest touches the ground, or very close to it, push back up to the starting position.

Crunches

Crunches tone your abdominal muscles. They don't require any equipment other than a mat, carpet, or towel to protect your back.

Lie down on your back with your knees bent and your feet flat on the ground. Place your hands behind your head and press your lower back into the mat. From there, lift your shoulders off the ground and curl your upper body towards your knees.

Reverse the motion and repeat. No need to rush; the slower the better!

Lunges

To perform a lunge, start by standing upright with your feet hip-width apart. Take a step forward with one foot, keeping your torso straight and your shoulders back and relaxed. Look straight ahead. Lower your body by bending your front knee to about a 90-degree angle, while the back knee hovers just above the ground. Make sure your front knee is directly above your ankle and doesn't push out too far. Push back up through the heels, and return to your starting position. Repeat this motion on the other side. Focus on maintaining good form to avoid strain or injury.

And of course, don't forget **The Commuter's Workout**. If your workplace or grocery store is nearby, consider walking or cycling instead of driving. You can achieve a moderate-intensity workout and do a favour for the planet at the same time.

Yoga, Tai Chi, and Pilates

All three disciplines, while distinct in their own right, overlap in their holistic approach to well-being, blending physical exercise with mental clarity. I can strongly recommend all three of these.

Yoga

Yoga is an age-old practice originating from ancient India. It offers an intricate combination of postures, breathing techniques, and meditation. Yoga doesn't merely promote flexibility and muscle strength, but also fosters mental tranquillity. Research shows a positive correlation between yoga and improved cardiovascular health, alongside reduced stress levels and enhanced cognitive function (Woodyard, 2011).

Tai Chi

Tai Chi is a Chinese martial art practised for both its defensive training and health benefits. This gentle form of exercise emphasises fluid movements and deep breathing, offering numerous health benefits such as improved balance, flexibility, cardiovascular health, and even a decrease in stress and anxiety (Harvard Health Publishing, 2019).

Pilates

Pilates, described as a 'mind-body intervention', is a comprehensive fitness method created in the early 20th century by physical trainer Joseph Pilates. This practice focuses on the core postural muscles that aid in keeping the body balanced and provide support for the spine. Pilates has a strong emphasis on proper alignment, control, breathing, flowing motion, and developing a strong core or *powerhouse*. It integrates the body with the mind, enhancing focus, muscular control, precision, and whole-body awareness. Whether you're a fitness novice or a seasoned athlete, Pilates offers a potent, adaptable approach to well-being, improving physical strength, flexibility, balance posture and endurance. Many people report an increase in concentration and improvements in stress management.

For all three disciplines, look for beginner's classes in your local area, or find a certified instructor who can guide you through the fundamentals. You could also consider online classes if in-person options aren't available. The beauty of all these practices is their adaptability; they can be customised to suit any fitness level, from beginners to seasoned practitioners. Incorporating these disciplines into your weekly routine alongside the DASH diet can cultivate a holistic approach to your health journey and offer many benefits.

It is recommended to start with short, manageable sessions, gradually increasing the duration as you grow more comfortable. Consistency is key; every bit of movement counts towards your health goals.

Chapter Summary

Physical activity has numerous benefits, including weight management, cardiovascular health, improved mood, and enhanced energy levels. Importantly, exercise can further lower blood pressure, making it an excellent complement to the DASH diet, which is designed with the primary aim of reducing hypertension.

By including regular exercise in your daily routine, you will increase the speed at which weight loss occurs. Different types of exercise will bring about different results, but ultimately you will be burning calories and increasing your muscle mass.

The most crucial point is to find an exercise routine you enjoy and can stick with it. Pick something that complements your personality and lifestyle. By doing so, you will be able to make this a far more sustainable option for you, allowing you to enjoy lasting benefits from this new way of healthy living. Make sure you're engaging in physical activity regularly. Physical activity should be a pleasure, not a chore.

I encourage you to delve into my bonus book, 'DASH Diet 30-Minute Workouts'. This resource contains further information, with practical examples of workout and exercise routines you can do comfortably at home. Access the book at:

https://amitylifebooks.com/dashfree

Chapter 4: Combining the DASH Diet and Exercise

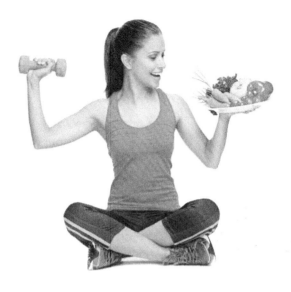

"We cannot start over. But we can begin now and make a new ending."

—Zig Ziglar[5]

As we embark on this next chapter, let it be known that this part might be shorter than you might expect. Not because it's any less important—quite the contrary. But simply because you already have all the tools at your disposal. You now have the knowledge, strategies, and examples needed to start this life-changing journey. What remains now is action—your action!

This chapter serves as a launching pad rather than an information hub, nudging you to take that pivotal step. It

---

[5] American author and motivational speaker

encourages you to synthesise everything you've learned so far and incorporate it into your life. Success isn't merely about acquiring knowledge; it's about applying it. So, brace yourself, and let's take this next step together towards a healthier, happier life with the DASH diet and regular exercise.

Understanding the Relationship Between Diet, Exercise, and Metabolism

To achieve optimal weight loss, energy expenditure through exercise must be combined with a reduction in caloric intake, which is where the DASH diet comes in. But balancing a regular exercise routine with the DASH diet presents an **optimal approach** towards healthy weight loss. The combination of exercise and diet is also important for **long-term weight maintenance**. The DASH diet's nutrient-rich, balanced approach can also help regulate blood sugar levels and maintain a steady energy supply, again required for physical activity. It's a win-win combination.

Combining exercise with DASH is about cultivating a lifestyle that promotes well-being and vitality. This lifestyle will require effort and commitment, but the rewards—better health, improved energy, and a sense of accomplishment—are well worth it. Stay motivated and stay consistent.

Setting Realistic Goals — Realism Reigns, Fantasy Wanes

In the realm of fitness, health and diet—weight loss included— success is not determined by the speed of your progress, but by the **consistency** of your efforts. Setting realistic goals is the cornerstone of any long-lasting change.

A realistic weight loss goal is typically about 1 to 2 pounds per week. This rate is generally achievable with a combination of regular physical activity and a healthy diet that creates a caloric deficit of between 500 to 1,000 calories per day. Noting that the 1,000 calories a day deficit is at the very top end of what is approaching 'rapid weight loss'.

As everyone's body responds differently to weight loss efforts, it's crucial to set goals that promote a healthy and sustainable lifestyle change rather than simply focusing on the numbers on the scale. Some may find their weight loss journey includes periods of weight stability or slower loss, and that's okay. The ultimate goal should always be improved health and wellness.

To achieve the calorie deficit, we have set out above, we need to set **realistic** and **achievable** diet and fitness goals. These goals should be Specific, Measurable, Achievable, Relevant, and Time-bound, often referred to as SMART goals.

For example, a SMART goal for exercise could be: "I will walk briskly for 30 minutes, five days a week, for the next four weeks." This goal is **specific** (walk briskly), **measurable** (30 minutes, five days a week), **achievable** and **realistic** (assuming baseline fitness allows for brisk walking), relevant (it promotes health and contributes to weight loss), and **time-bound** (for the next four weeks).

A SMART goal for following the DASH diet could be: "I will follow the DASH diet plan with a focus on consuming 4 servings of fruits and vegetables, 6 servings of grains, 2 servings of low-fat or non-fat dairy, and lean proteins every day". This goal is **specific**; "I will keep a detailed food diary to monitor the daily intake from the food groups". This is **measurable**. "I will begin by incorporating these food groups into each meal". This is **achievable** by adding more vegetables to lunch and dinner meals, and switching from whole milk to low-fat milk. This goal is **relevant**, as it aligns with the overall health objective of improving nutrient intake. It is promoting weight loss and enhancing heart health. "I will commit to consistently meeting these dietary targets within a one-month timeframe, after which I will evaluate and adjust the plan accordingly". This makes the goal **time-bound**.

While the goal you set may seem challenging at times, the benefits that it will bring make every effort worthwhile. Take some time now to write down **your** goal now. Make it SMART.

The 7 Day Blueprint

Well, here we are. Let's combine everything we've learnt up to this point. This plan is ideal for **beginners**.

Day 1:

- **Breakfast:** Oatmeal topped with a handful of mixed berries and a teaspoon of honey.

- *Exercise:* 30-minute brisk walk around your neighbourhood.

- **Lunch:** Grilled chicken salad with mixed greens.

- *Exercise:* 15 minutes of light stretching or yoga poses.

- **Dinner:** Shrimp stir-fry with a variety of vegetables and a serving of brown rice.

- *Exercise:* Dance to your favourite music for 20 minutes to get your heart rate up.

Day 2:

- **Breakfast:** Two boiled eggs with a slice of whole-grain toast.

- *Exercise:* 30 minutes of bodyweight exercises like push-ups, squats, and lunges.

- **Lunch:** Tuna salad wrapped in whole grain tortillas.

- *Exercise:* 15 minutes of yoga or Pilates.

- **Dinner:** Baked chicken breast with a side of quinoa salad.

- *Exercise:* 30-minute bike ride (or use a stationary exercise bike).

Day 3:

- **Breakfast:** Greek yoghurt with a sprinkle of granola and a handful of blueberries.

- *Exercise:* 30-minute jog or brisk walk.

- **Lunch:** Quinoa Salad with Roasted Vegetables.

- *Exercise:* 15-minute yoga or tai chi session.

- **Dinner:** Turkey and quinoa stuffed bell peppers.

- *Exercise:* 30 minutes of dancing or a light aerobics routine.

Day 4:

- **Breakfast:** Whole grain cereal with skim milk and a banana.

- *Exercise:* 30 minutes of brisk walking or marching in place.

- **Lunch:** Greek salad with grilled chicken.

- *Exercise:* 15 minutes of stretching or Pilates.

- **Dinner:** Zucchini noodles with pesto and cherry tomatoes.

- *Exercise:* 30-minute stationary bike ride or simulate bicycling while lying on your back.

Day 5:

- **Breakfast:** Veggie scrambled eggs with a side of whole grain toast.

- *Exercise:* 30-minute session of bodyweight exercises like push-ups, squats, and lunges.

- **Lunch:** Turkey sandwich with whole grain bread and a side of mixed greens.

- *Exercise:* 15 minutes of light yoga or tai chi.

- **Dinner:** Baked salmon with lemon and dill, served with a side of roasted vegetables.

- *Exercise:* 30 minutes of dancing or light aerobics routine.

Day 6:

- **Breakfast:** Smoothie made with spinach, banana, blueberries, and skim milk.

- *Exercise:* 30-minute jog.

- **Lunch:** Chickpea and vegetable curry served with a side of brown rice.

- *Exercise:* 15-minute stretching or Pilates.

- **Dinner:** Vegetable stir-fry with tofu.

- *Exercise:* 30-minute stationary bike ride or simulate bicycling while lying on your back.

Day 7:

- **Breakfast:** Greek yoghurt topped with a handful of mixed berries and a sprinkle of granola.

- *Exercise:* 30 minutes of brisk walking or marching in place.

- **Lunch:** Tuna salad with mixed greens.

- *Exercise:* 15-minute yoga or tai chi session.

- **Dinner:** Grilled chicken salad with mixed greens.

- *Exercise:* 30 minutes of dancing or light aerobics routine.

Again, more repetition here, but finding the right **balance** between diet and exercise is critical for sustainable weight loss and health improvement. This balance is also critical for long-term weight maintenance.

This is **your** plan, so adapt it as you see fit. Aim for a good night's sleep after each, and listen to your body to avoid overexertion.

Dash Challenges

Embarking on the DASH diet may bring its own set of challenges, particularly if it is just you who will be adopting the diet. It's important to recognise these potential challenges and prepare for them.

- **The Lone Dasher:** If it's only you who will be following the DASH diet, you might face challenges during mealtimes, or feel tempted by others eating non-DASH food. This requires self-discipline and the ability to stay committed to your health goals even when others around you aren't on the same journey.

- **The Family DASH:** If you're planning to get your whole family on board, remember that everyone might not be as enthusiastic about the changes as you are. Sit everyone down and explain the benefits of the diet, and how it can help the whole family become healthier. Create meal plans that are exciting and appealing to all family members to encourage participation. Incorporating 'DASH Days' may help with this.

- **Dashing for Someone Else:** If you're implementing the DASH diet for someone else, such as an elderly parent or a child, there could be resistance. Approach this delicately, stressing the health benefits and showing support and patience as they adjust to the new eating style.

Difficult conversations can arise when explaining why you're choosing healthier options, dealing with potential resistance, or declining certain foods. Be ready to explain your reasons and hold your ground, reminding yourself and others that this is about health and well-being.

Change may be challenging, but not impossible.

Blood Pressure Log

Keeping a detailed blood pressure log is an indispensable step for those adopting this diet and lifestyle if it is primarily to manage hypertension. Keeping a blood pressure log can be highly beneficial for several reasons:

- **Monitoring trends:** Monitoring your readings can provide a clearer picture of your progress and aid in the effective management of your condition. It also helps both you, and your healthcare provider, identify patterns and trends over time.

- **Evaluating treatment effectiveness:** If you are on medication for high blood pressure, a log can provide valuable feedback on whether the treatment plan is working or if adjustments are needed (in consultation with your doctor).

- **Understanding triggers:** By noting what activities, foods, or stressors precede a blood pressure reading, you can better understand what may be causing fluctuations and work on strategies to mitigate these triggers.

- **Improving communication with your doctor:** Bringing a blood pressure log to your appointments can facilitate more productive conversations. It provides a clear, tangible overview of your health data that can inform treatment decisions.

- **Promoting responsibility:** Keeping a log can increase your sense of ownership and responsibility over your health. This will encourage more proactive habits and mindfulness about lifestyle choices that impact blood pressure.

There is a Blood Pressure Log ready for you to print out and use. Download it for free at:

https://amitylifebooks.com/dashfree

The Power of Sleep

It is well-known that diet and sleep are two important pillars of health. In fact, they are inextricably linked. Both play a role in our overall well-being and how our bodies function. When it comes to weight loss, sleep may be more important than you think.

Many studies show that people who sleep less are more likely to be overweight, or obese, than those who sleep a healthy seven to eight hours a night. Researchers believe that this is because sleep deprivation leads to changes in hormones that increase hunger and cravings for unhealthy foods which impacts maintaining a healthy weight (Boston and Ma). In addition, when you're tired, you're more likely to make poor food choices and have less energy to exercise. All of these factors can sabotage your weight-loss efforts. Sleep has many benefits, including:

- Building up your immunity.

- Reducing your likelihood of developing significant health issues like diabetes and heart disease.

- Reducing stress and improving your mood.

- Improving your ability to think clearly and perform your duties better.

- Making good decisions and avoiding accidents. This becomes more important when we add exercise into the mix.

The bottom line is, if you're trying to lose weight, make sure you're getting enough sleep. Aim for seven to eight hours of regular, good quality sleep per night. And if you have trouble sleeping, talk to your doctor about possible solutions.

Healthy Choices — In Sight, and In Mind

I've incorporated this segment into this chapter, as I genuinely believe it carries significant importance. We all know that healthy eating is important for our overall health and well-being, but sometimes it's hard to make healthy choices. This can often happen when we are on the go, out and about, or where healthy options are not readily available. By having a ready supply of healthy food within reach, we are less likely to make bad choices about what we eat. Moreover, when we are not snacking on unhealthy foods, we are more likely to maintain a healthy weight and stick to our goal.

Foods that you are drawn to in times of stress should be replaced with healthy alternatives. Some ideal healthy options include dried fruits, nuts and seeds. By keeping these kinds of foods on hand, you will be more likely to reach for them when you are feeling hungry. This one simple change could make all the difference in maintaining a healthy lifestyle.

Following Recipes — Guesswork is Not an Ingredient!

There are a number of 'weight loss recipes' available, and it can be difficult to know which ones are right for you, or indeed right at all. Not all recipes are created equal, and some may actually be not quite as healthy as we would like.

Once you have found a recipe that you feel comfortable with, the next step is to actually follow it correctly. This means not only using the right ingredients, but also measuring them out correctly. This can be difficult, especially if you are not used to cooking with measurements. However, it is important to make sure that you follow the recipe exactly in order to get the best results. Don't be tempted to add extra ingredients.

If you are having trouble finding weight loss recipes that work for you, there are a number of trusted resources available online. You can also ask your friends at the gym, or indeed anyone who seems to have a grasp of fitness and health. Asking family members for their favourite recipes may not always result in the healthiest of choices. Whatever route you choose, make sure that you find a recipe that you feel comfortable with, and that will help you to achieve your weight loss goals.

Chapter Summary

Integrating regular physical activity into your lifestyle is a crucial component to augment the benefits of the DASH diet. In this chapter, we've delved into the intersection of the DASH Diet and exercise. We introduced a detailed 7-day plan, designed with a balance of nutrient-dense meals and manageable exercises. We also discussed practical strategies to navigate potential challenges that may arise. In the next chapter, we will cover everything you need to ensure success with your SMART goal.

Chapter 5: Staying the Course

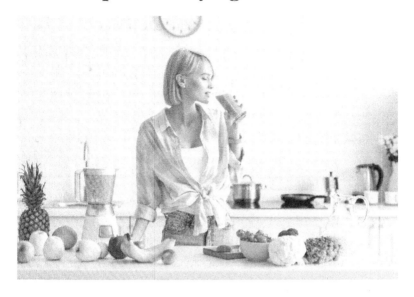

"If you want to be happy, set a goal that commands your thoughts, liberates your energy and inspires your hopes."

—Andrew Carnegie[6]

Whatever your goal may be, success is only achieved when it is met. You should hopefully have your SMART goal (or goals!) written down from chapter 4, or have a goal placed firmly in your mind. There are many factors that will contribute to you achieving this goal. There are also factors that may prevent you from reaching it. In this chapter, we will learn about these factors, and how they may apply to you.

---

[6] Scottish-American industrialist and philanthropist.

Keep Thoughts Positive

When following any new health venture, it is important to keep your thoughts positive. Research has shown that people who allow negative thoughts to control, or creep into their thinking and actions are more likely to give up on their goal. This could mean returning to unhealthy food, stopping exercise or regaining the weight that has been lost. Whereas people who focus on positive thoughts, are more likely to stay the course, and achieve their goals.

One way to keep your thoughts positive is to focus **only** on the positive results you will achieve. For example, think about how good you will look and feel once you reach your goal. Think of the benefits that a healthy diet and exercise will bring with it.

It is easier to stay positive if you set realistic goals. For example, don't set a goal that involves losing too much weight too quickly. As well as being not well advised, it will be difficult to sustain, and discouraging, if you fail. Instead, aim to lose a modest amount of weight over time, and celebrate each small victory along the way.

Negative thinking can also lead to a physical response and cause stress, which can sometimes lead to headaches and fatigue. When stress hormones are released into the body, they can put you at risk of developing other health problems. This not only makes life difficult, but it can affect your mental state.

Everyone makes mistakes sometimes. If you slip up and eat something unhealthy, don't beat yourself up about it. Just get back on track the next day. This lifestyle is for the long term, and one mistake will not undo all your hard work.

Visualise Success

You may have been taught the technique of putting your primary aim or objective in writing and sharing this goal with others. This is definitely a good practice and can be beneficial in achieving a goal you have set yourself. However, visualisation goes further. Visualisation is actually picturing yourself, not only achieving your goal, and how this will make you feel, but also visualising in your mind getting to that goal. This process should include visualising all the obstacles you may encounter along your way and how you will overcome them if they arise. This powerful technique is proven to enhance your chances of success and reduce any anxiety you may be feeling.

To do this, start by thinking about how you will achieve your goal with DASH and exercise. What is required? What are the probable challenges that you might face? Use a pen and a piece of paper to do this now and record your thoughts. Think about your primary objective, and set a timeline, preferably one that is not too long. An example might be "I want to lose one stone of weight. To do this, I will lose one pound a week for fourteen weeks". For every potential obstacle you can think of, start thinking and visualising how you might overcome these. An example could be, "We always eat out at the weekend; how can I still stick to my goal?". In visualising everything before you start, you have already imagined what could happen in your mind, and when it does in reality, you will be prepared.

Spend a few moments each day visualising yourself achieving your goals. This will help keep you motivated and focused.

Do not underestimate this technique. Visualisation will help you reach your goals, no matter what they are.

Saying NO To Food Pushers

We all know them. The food pushers. The ones who are always trying to get us to eat more, or try different food, or both! They're the ones who are always talking about food, and how good it is, and how we should try it. And they're usually right—the food is good. But that doesn't mean we want to eat it all the time, or that we need to.

So why do they do it? Well, there are a few possible reasons. First, some people just love food. They're passionate about it, and they want to share that passion with others. Second, some people see food as a way to bond with others. They think that if they can get us to eat more, or try new things, then we'll be closer to them. And lastly, some people may just be trying to help. They think that if we eat more, then we'll be happier. Again, this can be true for some of us, some of the time, but sometimes our relationship with food can be our undoing.

Often it looks like it's coming from a good place, but it can be a violation of boundaries, especially if it involves making remarks about eating preferences, or trying to pressure you into having something you don't want. Whether it's deliberate or not, the pressure to be polite can leave you feeling uneasy and possibly derail any positive changes you're trying to make.

Regardless of the reason, it can be frustrating to deal with food pushers. But there are a few ways to handle them. First, you can try to politely decline their offer. This can be difficult, especially if they're insistent, but it's worth a try. Second, you can **explain** your own eating habits and preferences. This may help them understand where you're coming from, and why you don't want to eat what they're offering.

So next time you are faced with a food pusher, remember that you have options. You don't have to eat what they're offering, and you don't have to put up with their prodding. Just politely decline, explain yourself, or walk away. You are in charge of what you put in your body, and you aren't required to provide anyone with reasons for why you do what you do.

Overcoming Tiredness

Starting a diet, especially one that may involve a reduction in calories can initially lead to feelings of tiredness. This is often due to your body adjusting to obtaining energy from different sources, especially if you are used to a diet of high sugar or high fat foods.

Exercise, particularly when you're starting a new routine, can also lead to fatigue as your body is being pushed beyond its usual routine. However, this typically improves over time as your strength and endurance increase. In fact, regular exercise is known to boost energy levels in the long term. As your body becomes fitter and stronger, you'll have more stamina for daily activities.

To manage your energy levels during this transition period, it's important to ensure your diet is well-balanced and nutritious. Consuming whole, nutrient-dense foods can provide you with sustained energy. Hydration is also crucial; dehydration can lead to fatigue, whereas good hydration will help your body to function optimally. Proper rest is equally important. Make sure you're getting enough sleep every night, as sleep is essential for muscle recovery and energy restoration. When you are well-rested, your body will have more energy to devote to metabolism.

You may find that eating smaller, more frequent meals rather than 2 or 3 large meals, is helpful. This will help your body to better digest the food you are eating and prevent blood sugar crashes that lead to fatigue. Talking of which, don't give in to processed foods and sugary snacks. Yes, these will give you a quick burst of energy, but will quickly fade and leave you feeling even more tired.

If everything is going to plan, as your body adapts to your new diet and exercise regimen, you will see an overall improvement in your energy levels. If persistent fatigue, or drastic changes in energy levels occur, it may be best to consult with a healthcare professional to rule out any underlying condition.

Dining Out and Taking Vacations

Dining out and taking vacations should not derail your healthy lifestyle and weight loss efforts. While these situations present unique challenges, they can be managed effectively with proper planning and strategic choices.

Dining Out

Dining out when you are on a diet can be tricky. You want to enjoy your food, but you also want to make sure you are getting the nutrients your body needs. It's all about making smart choices and controlling portion sizes. Always consider the DASH dietary principles and choose dishes that are low in sodium and rich in fruits, vegetables, lean proteins, and whole grains.

Here are some tips for eating healthy food when dining out:

- If you get any say in the matter (!), choose a restaurant that more or less caters to your diet.

- Choose grilled, broiled, or steamed options over fried or sautéed dishes. Avoid dishes with cream or cheese sauces, which can be high in sodium and saturated fat.

- Look for salads or other vegetable-based dishes on the menu. When ordering, ask for the dressing on the side and use it sparingly. Restaurant salad dressings can be high in sodium and added sugars.

- Don't be shy about making special requests. Restaurants are accustomed to accommodating dietary needs these days. Ask for sauces on the side, request that your dish be prepared with less salt, or ask for a side of steamed vegetables instead of fries. Ask about the ingredients in a dish **before** ordering to make sure that you are not consuming too much fat, sugar, or salt.

- You may have noticed that meal portion sizes have grown over the years, with restaurant portions being often larger than what you might serve at home. Consider sharing a meal or taking half of it home for another meal to avoid overeating.

Vacations

When on vacation, maintaining your exercise routine can be a bit more challenging, but it is far from impossible. Just because you're on vacation doesn't mean you have to abandon your healthy eating habits! There are plenty of ways to enjoy your holiday without overindulging, and incorporating physical activity into your vacation can even enhance your holiday. Here are some tips and things to think about:

- Think about the things that may make it hard to stick to your plan and prepare a strategy for dealing with them. The main issues may be alcohol, snacks, and extras, social pressure and serving sizes. Keep your goals in mind. Decide whether the goal is to simply prevent weight gain during your holiday, or active continued loss.

- If it's a road trip, or a long journey, make sure to pack healthy snacks and meals for the trip. This way, you can avoid unhealthy options at airports or restaurants.

- Choose vacations that inherently involve physical activities. This can be as simple as sightseeing on foot or bicycle, opting for a hiking adventure, or even trying a new sport or activity. If they have one, use the hotel gym or pool. If your accommodations include these facilities, take full advantage of it.

- Consider your usual alcohol consumption while you're on vacation, and think about how you're going to manage that.

The Dreaded Weight Plateau

If you've been following a weight loss plan but have recently hit a plateau, don't despair. It's common for people to experience a weight loss plateau at some point. Here are a couple of things you can do to overcome this and continue on your path to success.

- Take a close look at your diet and make sure you're still eating the right foods and serving recommendations. It's easy to slip into old habits when you're not seeing the results you want. Zero-fat yoghurt quickly becomes low-fat, which graduates to high-fat! The same is true with bread, pasta and rice, going from brown to white. It's going to be the staples that will creep up on you, rather than a cake binge.

- Up your exercise routine. If you've been sticking to the same workout routine, try adding some new exercises or increasing the intensity of your workouts. This will help jumpstart your metabolism and get things moving again.

Don't get discouraged. A weight loss plateau is not a sign that you're not doing well. Stay positive and keep up the good work and you'll eventually reach your goals.

Understanding the Vegetarian Diet

When it comes to weight loss, a vegetarian diet can be extremely effective. Studies have shown that following a vegetarian diet can help you lose weight, and keep it off. For those among you who have made the switch to plants, to answer your question; Yes! You can definitely combine the vegetarian diet with the DASH diet. In fact, the combination can be very beneficial, as both diets emphasise the consumption of fruits, vegetables, whole grains, and legumes. The DASH diet specifically aims to lower sodium intake and promote heart health, while a vegetarian diet avoids meat and often results in lower overall calorie consumption. With some planning and mindful selection of plant-based proteins and nutrient-dense foods, it's absolutely possible to adhere to both diets simultaneously.

There are several reasons why a vegetarian diet is so effective for weight loss. First, vegetarians typically eat fewer calories than those who eat meat. Second, plant-based foods are generally lower in fat and calories than animal-based foods. Third, a vegetarian diet is, more often than not, rich in fibre, which can help you feel full and satisfied after meals. Fourth, many vegetables are naturally low in sodium, which can help reduce water retention and bloating.

On the flip side of all this, while the DASH diet does emphasise the consumption of fruits, vegetables, and whole grains, it doesn't require you to fully embrace vegetarianism. This dietary approach accommodates various sources of lean protein, such as poultry, fish, and low-fat dairy, which are all part of a balanced, non-vegetarian diet. Therefore, whether you're a meat lover, pescatarian, or flexitarian, you can certainly adopt and benefit from the principles of the DASH diet.

If you're considering switching to a vegetarian diet for weight loss, it's important to make sure you're getting all the nutrients your body needs, particularly protein and vitamin B12, which are commonly derived from animal products. In addition to consuming an abundance of fruits, vegetables, whole grains and legumes, vegetarians can find a rich source of protein in many alternatives like beans, tofu, lentils and nuts.

Understanding the Vegan Diet

There are many reasons why individuals might choose to follow a vegan diet. Some base their decision on grounds believing that all animals should be treated with compassion and respect; I agree. Others advocate veganism on environmental or health concerns; a worthy cause indeed. Regardless of the motivation, it is important to understand the principles of what is involved in a vegan diet and to ensure that if you do decide to follow it, that you are getting all the nutrients that your body needs.

The most obvious principle of the vegan diet is that it excludes **all animal products** such as meat, poultry, fish, eggs, dairy products and honey. This means that vegans must seek other sources for their nutrients. Similar to the vegetarian diet approach, it is vital to consume a range of plant based foods in order to fulfil this. As well as protein and vitamin B12; iron, calcium and omega-3 fatty acids also become elements which are commonly found in animal products.

When adapting the DASH diet into a vegan lifestyle, you should replace animal proteins with plant-based alternatives, like lentils, chickpeas tofu, tempeh or seitan. Additionally, nuts and seeds can replace dairy as a source of healthy fats. Fortified plant milks, flaxseeds, chia seeds, almonds, walnuts and nutritional yeast all help ensure adequate intake of nutrients. As always, it's best to consult a registered dietitian or healthcare provider when significantly changing your diet to ensure all nutritional needs are being met.

Fibre

Fibre plays an instrumental role in weight loss, and it's an essential part of the DASH diet. Fibre-rich foods tend to be more filling, so you're likely to eat less and stay satisfied for longer. Consuming adequate fibre can also aid in maintaining stable blood sugar levels, which is important in preventing insulin spikes that can lead to hunger and weight gain.

In the context of the DASH diet, high fibre foods such as whole grains, fruits, vegetables, and legumes are emphasised. These foods not only provide fibre but also a wealth of other nutrients. For example, a breakfast on the DASH diet might include a bowl of oatmeal topped with berries and a sprinkle of nuts, which is high in fibre and can help keep you satisfied until lunch. As with any dietary changes, it's recommended to increase fibre intake gradually to allow your body to adjust and to ensure you're also drinking plenty of water.

Here are some high-fibre foods that can easily be incorporated into the DASH diet to increase fibre intake.

- **Whole Grains:** Foods like whole grain bread, oatmeal, brown rice, and whole grain pasta are excellent sources of fibre.

- **Fruits:** Pears, apples, and bananas are high in fibre. Remember to eat the skin where a lot of the fibre can be found (not the banana skin though!). Remember to give all fruit a good wash.

- **Vegetables:** Broccoli, carrots, Brussels sprouts, and all types of squash have high fibre content.

- **Legumes:** Foods such as lentils, black beans, chickpeas are rich in fibre.

- **Seeds and Nuts:** Chia seeds, flax seeds, almonds, and pistachios are good sources of fibre.

- **Tubers:** Potatoes, sweet potatoes, and other tubers are high in fibre. Jacket potatoes are a quick and simply, high fibre meal.

- **Popcorn:** If it's air-popped and lightly seasoned (no salt or butter), popcorn can be a good source of fibre.

- **Avocados:** These are rich in fibre and healthy fats.

- **Berries and soft fruit:** Blackberries and raspberries are particularly high in fibre.

- **Dark Chocolate:** Choose a high-quality dark chocolate with a high percentage of cocoa, and it will be both delicious and relatively high in soluble fibre.

As always, aim for variety in your diet to ensure you're getting a wide range of nutrients. Eating 3 bars of dark chocolate in one sitting does not constitute a balanced approach!

A Scientific Look at Protein

Protein is an essential nutrient for the human body and is required for the growth and maintenance of all tissues, including muscle tissue. We often hear that protein plays a pivotal role in weight loss; "Carbs bad, protein good". But why is this? Let's look at the science:

- **Satiety:** Protein-rich foods take longer to digest and metabolise, which means you feel fuller for longer and less likely to snack between meals. In turn, this aids in reducing your overall caloric intake.

- **Thermic Effect of Food (TEF):** Protein has a significantly higher TEF compared to carbohydrates and fat. This means that when you consume protein, your body uses more energy (calories) to digest and metabolise it than it does when digesting other nutrients. It is estimated that about 20-30% of the calories in the protein you consume are actually used during the digestion and metabolism process itself. If you compare this to only 5-10% for carbohydrates, and 0-3% for fats, it is easy to see why high-protein diets can support weight loss.

- **Muscle preservation:** As previously mentioned, when you're losing weight, you want to ensure that it's fat you're losing, and not muscle. Eating an adequate amount of protein (for muscle growth) while on a calorie-restricted diet can help preserve lean muscle mass, while allowing for fat loss.

- **Gluconeogenesis:** Gluconeogenesis is a process your body undergoes to create glucose from non-carbohydrate sources. Going back to our car analogy, imagining your body as a car with glucose as its fuel. When you've run out of readily available glucose (fuel) from recently eaten carbohydrates, your body doesn't just stall out. Instead, it starts gluconeogenesis, which is akin to having a backup generator. This "generator" powers up and starts creating glucose from other fuel types such as amino acids (from proteins), lactate, and glycerol (from fats). Gluconeogenesis is a slow and somewhat labour-intensive process for the body. Rather than quickly spiking, and then dropping blood sugar levels, as rapid digestion of carbohydrates can do, gluconeogenesis produces glucose at a more gradual, consistent rate. This aids in appetite control and promotes a feeling of fullness. In turn, this supports weight loss, as it reduces the urge for frequent snacking on high-calorie foods.

- **Hormonal regulation:** Protein-rich diets can regulate the levels of beneficial weight-controlling hormones. They reduce levels of the hunger hormone ghrelin, and boost the appetite-reducing hormones GLP-1, peptide

YY, and cholecystokinin. This leads to a reduction in calorie intake.

While protein is important for weight loss, it's crucial to obtain your protein from healthy sources like lean meats, fish, legumes, nuts, and whole grains, especially when following a diet like the DASH diet. Also, balance is key. Despite the importance of protein, a balanced intake of all macronutrients (carbohydrates, fats, and protein) is necessary for overall health and sustainable weight loss.

You should aim to get about 18% of your daily calories from protein when following DASH. If you are trying to lose weight, adding more protein to your diet can help you achieve your goals. Try incorporating some high-protein foods into your meals and snacks. For example, add a hard-boiled egg to your salad at lunch or have a low-fat yoghurt for a snack. The humble pea is a fantastic source of protein and can be added to salads, soups, rice dishes; the list goes on.

Keeping a Weight Loss Journal

If you're struggling to stick to your diet or exercise plan, maintaining a weight loss journal could be beneficial. It can help you identify any patterns that may be causing deviations from your plan. Once these patterns are recognised, you can make adjustments to your diet and exercise routine in order to avoid them in the future. Additionally, a weight loss journal serves as a tool for tracking progress and gauging **how well you're doing**. By monitoring your progress, it provides a representation of how far you've come and how much more effort is needed; a motivator if you like, allowing you to record your journey towards success.

When it comes to weight loss journals, there is an array of options available. There are journals specifically designed for weight loss, or you could simply use a notebook. Alternatively, there are numerous online platforms that offer journals tailored for this purpose. Regardless of the option chosen, just make sure it is quick and simple.

If you are going down the DIY route, to assist with entries, consider **honestly** answering some of the following questions:

1. What did I eat for breakfast, lunch, dinner, and snacks today?

2. How many glasses of water did I drink today?

3. Did I stick to my meal plan today? If not, what caused the deviation?

4. What physical activities or exercises did I do today?

5. How many hours of sleep did I get last night?

6. How did I feel before, during, and after my workouts?

7. On a scale of 1-10, how was my stress level today? What triggered my stress?

8. How am I feeling about my weight loss journey today?

9. What steps did I take to achieve my weight loss goals today?

10. What obstacles or challenges did I face today in adhering to my diet and exercise routine?

11. How can I overcome these challenges in the future?

12. Did I experience any cravings today? How did I handle them?

13. What are some small victories I can celebrate today?

14. What are three things I am grateful for today?

15. How can I make tomorrow even better and more aligned with my weight loss goals?

The answers to these questions can be very revealing. Just give it a go.

Do Something Else!

A parting piece of advice as we come to the end of this chapter is the importance of 'Doing Something Else'. It may seem out of place in 'how to' book about weight loss, but it's a tip that speaks volumes. This isn't about distraction or avoidance, but rather about the enrichment of your life.

Embarking on a diet and exercise regimen is undoubtedly important, but it's equally important to nurture your other interests and hobbies. Painting, playing a musical instrument, reading, writing, gardening, crafting, or volunteering in your local community—these activities do more than just fill your time. They enhance your mental well-being and provide a sense of accomplishment which compliments your weight loss journey.

Focusing solely on diet and exercise can sometimes lead to stress and obsession, which is counterproductive. By 'Doing Something Else', you're effectively diversifying your sources of happiness and fulfilment, which can actually enhance your motivation and perseverance in your weight loss efforts. It is a reminder that while you're working towards a healthier physical self, don't neglect the other aspects that make you, you.

Chapter Summary

In this chapter, we took an in-depth exploration of the complexities of sustaining your weight loss journey, emphasising the significance of consistency and commitment to the DASH diet and a regular exercise routine. We discussed the importance of setting realistic and achievable goals and overcoming common hurdles in your weight loss journey. This chapter highlighted practical strategies and provided useful tips on staying motivated. Enjoy the process, and most importantly, make your healthy lifestyle changes sustainable for long-term success. **Staying the course** is about perseverance, patience, and positivity in the face of challenges. It's about celebrating every victory, no matter how small, and constantly reminding yourself of your reason 'why'.

Chapter 6: Miscellaneous Tips, Tricks, Thoughts and Guidance

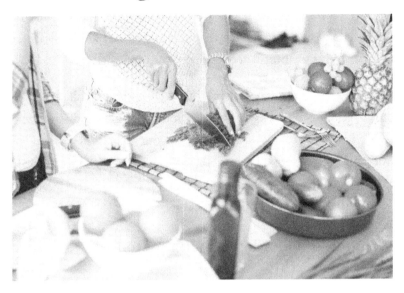

"Obstacles don't have to stop you. If you run into a wall, don't turn around and give up. Figure out how to climb it, go through it, or work around it."

—Michael Jordan[7]

You'll soon realise that the title of this chapter really does sum it up. This is the space where we delve into the wealth of knowledge, ideas, and strategies that I've picked up over the years whilst navigating the wonderful world of weight loss and exercise.

---

[7] Former professional basketball player and businessman

These nuggets of wisdom are all about the nitty-gritty of everyday living on the DASH diet. They may not fit neatly into any one topic, but they are far too important to be overlooked. From clever workout hacks that will motivate you to hit the gym, to practical diet advice that will make your DASH journey a breeze, this chapter is teeming with useful insights.

The beauty of this chapter is that it provides a wide range of ideas, leaving you free to pick something that resonates with you. So, open your mind, ready your highlighter (real or metaphorical), and dive into this cornucopia of handy DASH diet tips and tricks. You might just find the perfect piece of advice that makes everything click!

Alcohol — The Elephant in the Room

It's probably time we spoke about the elephant in the room—alcohol.

Alcohol is often referred to as 'empty calories' as it provides no nutritional benefit (other than carbs), yet contributes significantly to overall calorie intake. A single glass of wine or a bottle of beer can contain as many calories as a couple of pieces of sugary chocolate or a slice of pizza, and unfortunately, these calories don't make us feel full. What alcohol certainly does do is increase the likelihood of 'calorie overload'. What I mean by this is consuming your regular amount of calories, **plus extra** calories from alcohol. Consuming alcohol also increases the chances of making unhealthy food choices that often follow a few drinks, leading to yet more calories. This is a phenomenon which I am going to call, forever more, *'Liquor-Led Gluttony'*.

While moderate alcohol consumption can be a part of a balanced diet for many people, for others, it can become a hindrance to their health and fitness. For me personally, I decided to completely stop alcohol consumption 18 months ago. Now, I could say that this choice stemmed from recognising the impact alcohol had on my caloric intake, my sleep quality, or my overall energy levels. However, these are not the reasons. My primary motivation lay in the stark reality that I was unable to identify a single benefit of alcohol consumption. Moreover, the list of negatives could fill an entire book.

I realise that everyone's relationship with alcohol is personal and unique. What worked for me might not be the solution for you. It's crucial to find a balance that suits your lifestyle, preferences, and health goals. If you choose to drink, do so in moderation, and be aware of the effects it can have on your body, and your weight loss efforts. The DASH diet doesn't explicitly 'ban' alcohol. It defines moderation as drinking up to one drink per day for women and up to two drinks per day for men.

I believe it is simpler and more effective to stop alcohol consumption entirely. Even if this is just for however long you need it to be. This eliminates the need to worry about the extra calories, the potential impact on sleep quality, and the many other effects alcohol can have on the body. Going alcohol-free can bring about noticeable improvements in your health, fitness levels, and overall well-being **immediately**. Ultimately, however, the decision to stop drinking alcohol is a personal one and entirely up to you.

Intermittent Fasting (IF)

Intermittent fasting (IF) is a dieting approach that has gained substantial popularity in recent years. Unlike traditional diets, intermittent fasting does not specify what foods you should eat, but rather **when** you should eat them. IF is about establishing eating patterns that cycle between periods of eating and fasting.

The most common methods of IF include the 16/8 method, which involves fasting every day for 16 hours and restricting your daily eating window to 8 hours. Another is the 5:2 diet, where you consume only 500-600 calories on two non-consecutive days of the week, but then eat normally for the other five. It sounds complicated, but it isn't once you get into the swing of things.

Intermittent fasting has been heralded for its potential benefits, including weight loss, improved metabolic health, and even a longer life span. Some studies suggest it can help lower insulin levels, increase growth hormone levels, start cellular repair processes, and alter gene expression related to longevity and disease protection. That's a pretty impressive *curriculum vitae*.

The concept of intermittent fasting holds considerable promise and is a very broad topic that requires comprehensive exploration. To do IF justice would require an entirely separate book to delve into the specifics and how it can be effectively combined with other dietary approaches like the DASH diet. Watch this space—this is a current project of mine!

For the time being, it's important to note that while intermittent fasting can be an effective weight loss tool for some, it's not entirely suitable for everyone. This is particularly true for people with certain medical conditions, or pregnant women—for obvious reasons. If you're considering intermittent fasting, be sure to speak with your healthcare provider to first make sure it's right for you.

Vital Vitamins and Minerals for Weight Loss

Vitamins and minerals play key roles in weight loss and overall metabolic function. Here are a few to make note of:

- **Vitamin D:** Research indicates that individuals with adequate vitamin D levels tend to have healthier weights and are more successful in their weight loss efforts. Sun exposure and foods like fatty fish, cheese, and egg yolks all provide vitamin D.

- **B Vitamins:** The B vitamins, including B6, B12, and folic acid, play crucial roles in energy metabolism. They help the body metabolise carbohydrates, proteins, and fats, and use the stored energy in food. Foods rich in B vitamins include whole grains, meat, eggs, legumes, seeds, nuts, and dark leafy vegetables.

- **Iron:** Iron is essential for carrying oxygen to your muscles, helping them burn fat. Iron-rich foods include lean meats, shellfish, beans, and spinach.

- **Calcium:** Several studies have linked higher calcium intakes to lower body weights, and less weight gain over time. Dairy products are high in calcium, but let's not forget leafy greens and fortified foods like breakfast cereals.

- **Magnesium:** This mineral is necessary for energy production and can influence lipolysis; a process by which the body releases fat from its stores. Foods high in magnesium include whole grains, nuts, and green vegetables.

- **Zinc:** Zinc plays a key role in appetite control and therefore may also play a role in weight management. Research is ongoing. Foods rich in zinc include meat, shellfish, legumes, seeds, and dairy.

- **Vitamin C:** Vitamin C is a critical nutrient for the human body. It is involved in many biochemical processes, including the synthesis of collagen and the absorption of iron. Vitamin C is also a potent antioxidant, meaning it can help protect cells from damage caused by free radicals. A study published in the *American College of Nutrition Studies* stated that "Individuals with adequate vitamin C status oxidise 30% more fat during a moderate exercise bout than individuals with low vitamin C status; thus, vitamin C depleted individuals may be more resistant to fat mass loss." (Johnston). But let's be sensible here; guzzling litres of freshly squeezed orange juice will not make you lose weight. Quite the opposite, in fact! Again, balance is key.

- **Chromium:** Chromium plays a role in metabolising carbohydrates and fat. It is also necessary for proper insulin function. Dietary sources of chromium include broccoli, whole grains, nuts, seeds, lean meats, and some spices like cinnamon. You will note that many of the recipes in this book feature cinnamon.

- **Magnesium:** Magnesium is a mineral that's important for many bodily functions, including the regulation of blood sugar levels. It's also involved in energy metabolism and protein synthesis. Magnesium is found in a variety of foods, including green leafy vegetables, whole grains, nuts, and seeds.

Foods advocated by DASH provide a broad range of vitamins and minerals, such as the ones already mentioned. However, individual nutritional requirements vary based on a range of factors, including age, gender, physical activity level, medical history, and specific health goals. For some individuals, such as those with certain nutritional deficiencies or specific dietary restrictions, supplementing may be necessary. For instance, if you have a known deficiency in vitamin D or if you struggle to meet your calcium needs due to a dairy intolerance, a supplement would be a useful addition to your routine. If you don't fall into this bracket, you should be able to get everything you need from diet alone.

Smoothies and Juices

Smoothies and juices can be incorporated into a weight-loss plan, but they are not magic solutions for shedding unwanted pounds. The role they play in weight loss depends on their composition and how they are integrated into your **overall** diet.

Smoothies can be beneficial due to their highly satiating potential, while at the same time providing valuable nutrients. This is especially true when they are made with a balance of ingredients, such as fruits, vegetables, lean proteins (like Greek yoghurt), and healthy fats. They can serve as a meal. Notice that I've not used the word 'meal replacement' here. Smoothies should not 'replace' anything and should be 'stand-alone', containing all the nutrients your body requires, but in a convenient form. They work particularly well for breakfast!

Juices, on the other hand; while they provide a concentrated source of vitamins and minerals, they do lack the non-soluble fibre found in whole fruits and vegetables. They can also be high in sugar. Consuming too much juice can lead to excessive calorie intake, potentially hindering weight loss efforts.

Both smoothies and juices should be made primarily with vegetables, with fruits used sparingly to keep sugar content under control. Also, be aware of some store-bought versions. Some—but not all—come loaded with added sugars and lack the fibre, and full range of nutrients, found in homemade versions.

Up next is my go-to smoothie recipe. It packs in protein from the Greek yoghurt and almond (or peanut) butter, all of which are natural sources of protein. The addition of chia or flax seeds not only adds more protein, but also provides omega-3 fatty acids and fibre. Finally, the mixed berries and spinach give you a boost of vitamins and antioxidants, making this a nutrient-rich way to start your day. It's 100% DASH friendly.

They also make for an indulgent dessert, but watch those calories!

Nutty Banana-Berry Breakfast Smoothie

Ingredients:

- 1 cup mixed berries (strawberries, blueberries, raspberries). Frozen fruit also works well
- 1 medium ripe banana
- 1-2 tablespoons almond butter or peanut butter (look for low-sodium organic)
- 1/2 cup zero-fat Greek yoghurt (plain, unsweetened)
- 1 cup spinach
- 1 cup unsweetened almond milk or any other non-dairy milk
- 1 tablespoon chia seeds or flax seeds (or both)
- 1 teaspoon honey (optional)

Instructions:

1. Start by placing the almond milk in your blender.
2. Next, add the Greek yogurt, almond or peanut butter, banana, mixed berries, spinach, and the chia/flax seeds.
3. Blend all the ingredients together until smooth.
4. Taste, and if needed, add honey for extra sweetness and blend again.
5. Pour into a glass and enjoy!

Nutrition: Calories: 406, Protein: 15g, Fat: 14g, Carbs: 60g, Fibre: 13 g, Sodium: 247 mg

There are many different weight loss smoothie recipes available online and in cookbooks. Some of these recipes are more effective than others. In order to find the best recipe for your needs, consider the following:

- **The ingredients used in the recipe.** Make sure that the recipe uses healthy ingredients that promote weight loss, rather than weight gain. Avoid recipes that use sugary fruit juices or high-calorie mixers. Fruits with high sugar content include apples, grapes, mangos, oranges and pears.

- **The nutrition content of the recipe.** The recipe should be rich in vitamins and minerals in order to obtain the nutrients your body needs to lose weight.

- **The taste of the recipe.** The recipe should be palatable so that you will actually want to drink it. A Brussels sprout and cabbage smoothie may not be to your taste.

One of the latest trends in weight loss is "juice cleansing". This involves consuming nothing but fruit and vegetable juices for a period of time—usually three to seven days, and sometimes even longer. The basic idea behind this is to give your body a break from solid food, which allows it to "detoxify" and heal itself. Some people believe that this can help promote weight loss by resetting metabolism and aiding in digestion. However, there is no scientific evidence to support these claims. Furthermore, juice cleanses can be unsafe if not done "correctly". If you're considering a juice cleanse for weight loss, be sure to talk to your doctor first. This doesn't mean I'm not a fan of juicing—quite the opposite. It can be a fantastic way to consume lots of fruits and vegetables, especially when you're short on time. But consuming too much fruit juice can add extra calories and sugars to your diet, which can hamper weight loss efforts and spike your blood sugar levels. Care is required. Here are a few tips for sensible juicing:

- **Vegetable-focused juices:** Make vegetables the star of your juice. While fruits can add a dash of sweetness, they should not form the majority of your drink. This helps to keep sugar content in check.

- **No added sugars:** Fruit is already sweet, so avoid adding extra sugars or sweeteners. This includes "natural" sweeteners like honey or agave nectar. These sometimes help with smoothies, like my recipe above, but are not required in juices.

- **Portion control:** Even the healthiest of juices can add up in calories. Stick to small, controlled portions, generally 8 ounces or fewer.

- **Nutrition balance:** Don't rely on juices as your sole source of nutrition. Juices should be a supplement to a balanced diet, not a replacement.

- **Hydration:** Lastly, remember that while juices can contribute to your daily fluid intake, nothing replaces good old-fashioned water for hydration.

Canned Fish — No Fishing Trip Required

Canned fish is an option when it comes to a nutritious food that can support weight loss and overall health. It's packed with protein, aids in managing your appetite and promotes weight loss. The great thing about canned fish is its versatility and ease of use. Whether you're craving a salad, a light sandwich, or a savoury pasta dish, canned fish can easily be incorporated into your meal plan. Tuna, salmon, or sardines are all good choices. Canned fish is also rich in omega-3 fatty acids, which are essential for heart health. The convenience factor of canned fish is hard to beat; it has a long shelf life, and can be eaten directly from the can without any cooking required. Just remember to drain the can first!

There are some considerations to keep in mind when selecting canned fish though—especially if you follow the DASH diet. Some cautionary notes to keep in mind are:

- **Sodium content:** This is the big one. As we know; the DASH diet limits sodium intake, and unfortunately, canned fish, as a general rule, is high in sodium due to added salt. To reduce this risk, always buy "no salt added" or "low sodium". Rinsing canned fish under water before eating can help remove some excess sodium. Note, this is only possible when buying "in brine".
- **Mercury levels:** Some fish, such as tuna, can be high in mercury. This can pose a health risk when consumed in large amounts. It's advisable to limit consumption of high-mercury fish and instead choose lower-mercury

varieties like salmon and sardines. The elevated mercury content in tuna results from their diet, which consists of smaller fish that have already absorbed mercury from their environment. Light tuna, often skipjack, yellowfin or tongol, usually contains less mercury than white (albacore) tuna. So, when you're at the grocery store, choose cans labelled "light" over "white" or "albacore". Try to limit tuna intake to 2-3 servings per week or consider occasionally swapping out tuna for other types of canned fish. There are lots of varieties to choose from!

- **Packaging:** Fish packed in water tend to be lower in calories and unhealthy fats than those packed in oil. Choose water-packed options whenever available.

- **Sustainability:** Not really a diet concern, but certainly an ethical one—overfishing is a significant environmental concern. Look for brands that source their fish responsibly.

Weight Loss Vegetables

Where would I be without broccoli, cauliflower, beans and sweet potatoes? For many people, these vegetables are the key to achieving and maintaining weight goals.

- **Broccoli:** This cruciferous vegetable is low in calories and rich in fibre. It can also aid in digestion. Broccoli is packed with vitamins C, K, and A, along with other important minerals. Simple to cook and delicious.

- **Cauliflower:** Similar to broccoli, cauliflower is low in calories and high in fibre. It's a versatile vegetable that can be used as a low-carb substitute for grains and legumes in many dishes. Check out the Chilli Non Carne and Cauliflower Rice recipe in the next chapter!

- **Beans and Legumes:** These are an excellent source of protein and fibre, two key nutrients that can aid in weight management.

- **Sweet Potatoes:** These are high in dietary fibre, again, helping you feel fuller for longer and reducing calorie intake. They're also incredibly rich in vitamin A and provide a good amount of vitamin C, manganese, potassium, and several other key vitamins and minerals.

All of these vegetables can be easily incorporated into your DASH diet plan. Use them in soups, stews, salads, or side dishes, and you'll be adding a powerhouse of nutrition to your meals.

Soft Fruit

Soft fruits, such as berries, peaches, kiwis, and bananas, are a great addition to any diet, DASH or otherwise, and can play a significant role in weight loss and overall health:

- **Role in weight loss:** Soft fruits are low in calories and high in fibre. They also contain high levels of water, which adds to their weight-loss-friendly properties.

- **Ease of eating & no preparation:** One of the biggest advantages of soft fruits is their convenience. There's minimal preparation involved—just wash and eat. This makes fruit an easy go-to snack, especially when you're on the move, or short on time. Some soft fruits like bananas even come in their own biodegradable packaging.

- **Use in salads:** Soft fruits add a sweet and tangy punch to salads, making them more enjoyable. For example, strawberries can be used in a spinach salad, peaches in a chicken salad, or blueberries in a quinoa salad. This not only enhances the flavour profile but also adds an array of vitamins, minerals, and antioxidants. They look good too!

- **Nutritional value:** Soft fruits are packed with nutrients, including essential vitamins, minerals, and antioxidants that support overall health.

As well as having a high vitamin C content, berries in particular are rich in antioxidant phytonutrients known as Anthocyanins. Anthocyanins are a class of flavonoid that are responsible for the colour of many fruits and flowers. These pigments are also found in other plant-based foods, such as vegetables and tea. Anthocyanins have been shown to have various health benefits. By incorporating a variety of vibrant foods in your meals, you'll be well on your way towards maintaining a nutritious diet.

Similar to the advice on juicing—consume fruit as part of a balanced diet, and do not solely rely on them for weight loss.

Green Leafy Vegetables

Green leafy vegetables are more versatile than people think, and there is a common misconception that they are used solely in salads. They can be used in sauces, stews, and soups, or made into a delicious and healthy side dish by simply sauteing with a teaspoon of extra virgin olive oil and garlic. With the addition of lean protein, they can be easily transformed into a whole meal. Green leafy vegetables aid in weight loss efforts for several reasons:

- **Low in calories:** Green leafy vegetables, such as spinach, kale, lettuce, Swiss chard, and collard greens, are incredibly low in calories and high in fibre. This means you can pile on the salad without worrying about exceeding your daily calorie limit!

- **Nutrient-dense:** Green leafy vegetables are packed with a wide array of essential vitamins and minerals. They're particularly high in Vitamins A, C, K, and many of the B vitamins. They also provide minerals like iron, calcium, and potassium.

- **Antioxidant content:** Similar to fruit—vegetables are high in antioxidants which help fight inflammation in the body. Chronic inflammation has been linked to a variety of illnesses, as well as weight gain and obesity.

Healthy Dips — Where Veggies Find Their Perfect Match

I have a fondness for nutritious dips and they are great fun to make. Homemade dips, such as hummus, can support weight loss for several reasons:

- **Control over ingredients:** Making your own dips at home gives you the control over what goes into them. You can skip the high sodium and sugar content often found in store-bought versions.

- **Rich in fibre and protein:** Homemade hummus, which typically includes chickpeas, tahini (sesame seed paste), lemon juice, and garlic, is rich in fibre and protein. These ingredients promote feelings of satiety, helping to control appetite and prevent overeating.

- **Healthy fats:** Tahini and olive oil, common ingredients in hummus, are sources of monounsaturated and polyunsaturated fats. These types of fats, when consumed in moderation, can have a positive effect on heart health and help control weight.

Dips offer a range of possibilities and can be used in various ways. They can be spread on whole grain bread, used as dressings, for salads or enjoyed as dips with vegetables. These flavourful additions not only enhance the taste of meals but also encourage the consumption of more raw vegetables like carrots, celery and cucumber.

When it comes to calories, homemade hummus is a choice for those watching their intake. Compared to other dip options it is relatively low in calories. If you're looking to explore dip options and expand your repertoire, consider the following:

- Tzatziki—a refreshing Greek dip made from yogurt, cucumbers, garlic and fresh herbs like dill or mint. The high protein content in Greek yogurt makes this an excellent choice.

- Another option is salsa—a blend of tomatoes, onions, chillies and cilantro. Not only is salsa low in calories, but it also adds a burst of flavour to various dishes.

- For those who enjoy full on flavour, a roasted red pepper dip might be what you're looking for. By blending red peppers with garlic, tahini and a touch of vinegar; you create a deliciously vibrant dip.

- Guacamole—an all-time favourite that features ripe avocados mixed with lime juice. Often accompanied by tomatoes, onions and cilantro.

- Pesto is commonly used as a sauce but it can also serve as a dip. Made from basil, garlic, pine nuts and olive oil.

- Black Bean Dip is a hearty dip made from cooked black beans, garlic, cumin, and sometimes a splash of lime juice. Black beans are rich in protein and fibre.

- Baba Ghanoush is a creamy, smoky dip, made from roasted eggplants, tahini, lemon juice, and garlic. A good source of dietary fibre.

- Muhammara is a spicy dip originating from Syria. Made with walnuts, roasted red bell peppers, breadcrumbs, and pomegranate molasses. It's packed with flavours and has a complex texture.

Recipes for Baba Ghanoush, Muhammara and my personal Hummus recipe are included in the recipe section.

Probiotic and Prebiotic Foods

The digestive system is one of the most important systems in the human body. It is responsible for breaking down food and absorbing nutrients. Without a properly functioning digestive system, the body is unable to acquire the nourishment it needs. Probiotics and prebiotics have received a lot of attention for their benefits in maintaining gut health and overall well-being. Researchers are now exploring their impact on weight management, although the findings aren't entirely conclusive. Here are a few ways they may contribute to weight loss:

- Certain strains of probiotics can help restore balance to the gut by promoting the growth of beneficial bacteria linked to reduced fat storage and better appetite control.

- Probiotics may help strengthen the gut barrier, reducing the risk of inflammation related weight gain.

- Some specific probiotic strains have been found to influence the release of hormones like GLP 1 and PYY that play a role in controlling appetite.

- Several studies suggest that probiotics can limit the amount of fat absorbed in the intestines, resulting in its excretion, rather than storage.

- Prebiotics are components that are beneficial to gut bacteria fermentation. This fermentation process generates compounds that have the potential to enhance feelings of fullness, regulate blood sugar levels, and potentially boost metabolism.

- Prebiotics have the ability to enhance the absorption of minerals like calcium and magnesium, which play a role in fat metabolism.

Probiotic Foods:

- **Yogurt:** A well-known source of probiotics, particularly strains of Bifidobacterium and Lactobacillus. Having at least one serving per day will improve gut health and the immune function that is present within the digestive system. Yoghurt is delicious, and satisfying—it feels very indulgent when combined with honey. Raw honey is also a probiotic and prebiotic.

- **Kefir:** A fermented milk drink that contains an even wider variety of probiotic strains than yogurt.

- **Tempeh:** A fermented soy product originating from Indonesia. It's a great vegetarian meat substitute and is packed with probiotics.

- **Kombucha:** A fermented black or green tea drink. Now becoming very popular!

While incorporating probiotics into your diet can be beneficial for gut health, it's crucial to be mindful of the sodium content in certain probiotic-rich foods, particularly for those monitoring their blood pressure. Fermented foods like Sauerkraut, Kimchi, Miso, and certain types of fermented pickles often contain high levels of sodium content. This excessive sodium can raise blood pressure, counteracting the healthful intent of consuming these foods. While low-sodium alternatives may be available, it's essential to thoroughly check food labels and nutritional information.

Prebiotic Foods:

Prebiotics are types of dietary fibre that feed the friendly bacteria in your gut and help to stimulate the growth of beneficial microorganisms. Here are some of the best natural prebiotics:

- **Chicory Root:** Known for its coffee-like taste, it's a great source of the prebiotic fibre inulin.

- **Jerusalem Artichoke:** Not to be confused with regular artichokes. Jerusalem artichokes have properties similar to the potato but are different again. They contain around 15% of fibre by weight and can be enjoyed roasted, sautéed, or boiled.

- **Dandelion Greens:** Can be used in salads and are rich in fibre. Ask for these in all good organic health food shops.

- **Garlic:** About 10% of garlic's fibre content comes from inulin.

- **Onions:** Contain about 5% prebiotic fibre by weight and can be consumed raw (not for the faint-hearted!) or cooked.

- **Asparagus:** Delicious when grilled or roasted.

- **Bananas:** They contain small amounts of inulin and are also rich in resistant starch, especially when they're green.

- **Barley and Oats:** Both contain a large amount of the prebiotic fibre beta-glucan, which has been shown to promote healthy gut bacteria.

As with any dietary change, or when introducing any new foods into your diet, start slowly to give your gut time to adjust. If you are considering probiotics or prebiotics for weight loss purposes, understand that they are **one part** of the overall picture. DASH, with its full array of fruits, vegetables and whole grains will provide all your pre and probiotic needs without having to stress about whether you are lacking in this department.

Healthy Sweet Foods

Including healthy sweet foods in your diet can satisfy your sweet tooth and help to prevent overindulging in less healthy options. Consuming foods you enjoy, including the sweet ones, can give you a psychological lift and improve your mood; vital for maintaining long-term dietary changes. Healthy sweet foods contain natural sugars, which provide a quick source of energy, particularly beneficial before exercise. However, not so beneficial when eaten, minus the workout! Here are options for you to try:

- **Dates:** High in fibre, potassium, and various B vitamins, they are a great choice for a natural sweetener or a quick, energising snack. Buy good quality Medjool dates in bulk.

- **Apricots:** Dried apricots are an excellent source of vitamins A and E, as well as iron and potassium.

- **Raisins:** Raisins offer a quick dose of energy, and are rich in fibre, iron, and calcium.

- **Prunes:** Prunes, or dried plums, are well known for their fibre content and can aid in digestion.

- **Figs:** Dried figs are rich in fibre and provide a host of beneficial nutrients like magnesium, calcium, and potassium.

- **Cranberries**: Cranberries contain high levels of antioxidants and anthocyanins which are good for maintaining a healthy heart.

- **Goji berries:** These berries are packed with vitamins and minerals like vitamin C, fibre, iron, vitamin A, zinc and antioxidants.

- **Dried cherries:** Cherries have plenty of antioxidants and can help reduce inflammation.

- **Mulberries:** These berries are a powerhouse, rich in vitamin C, iron and calcium.

- **Mango:** Dried mango is particularly abundant in vitamin A.

Dried fruits are dense in nutrients but can also be high in sugars and calories due to their reduced water content. Always make sure to check the labels for added sugars before buying dried fruits.

Tea and Coffee

Tea is one of the most popular beverages worldwide and it can be a great addition to the DASH diet. It offers many health benefits and may even aid in weight loss. Besides keeping you hydrated, teas provide a range of antioxidants and other compounds that promote health. Green tea is especially known for its ability to boost metabolism. Research indicates that the compounds found in tea, such as flavonoids and caffeine, may have the potential to boost metabolism and encourage the burning of calories. This, in turn, could aid in weight loss. Some herbal teas, like hibiscus and chamomile, are naturally caffeine free. They also offer advantages such as improving sleep quality and aiding digestion. As we have learnt; both of these aspects play a role in weight management. Teas are not miracle workers though, and you should be cautious of any teas advertising themselves as such.

Similar to tea, coffee and its main active ingredient caffeine, has been linked to weight loss in various studies, primarily due to its potential effects on metabolism and fat burning. Research has suggested that caffeine may stimulate thermogenesis—the process by which the body generates heat and energy from digesting food. Caffeine can also enhance physical performance by mobilising fatty acids from the fat tissues to be used as an energy source.

While these findings indicate potential benefits of coffee (and tea) for weight loss, they should not be considered a definitive solution. These effects can vary greatly from person to person, and are often influenced by other lifestyle factors such as diet, physical activity, and overall health. The impact of caffeine on weight management is relatively small, and is typically short-lived as individuals often develop a tolerance to caffeine. The moral of the story is, don't expect caffeine to magically do all the work—as it won't.

Workout Hacks for the Home and Gym

Balancing work, family, personal life, and still finding time for exercise can be challenging. But exercise doesn't always have to be a time-consuming affair. Sometimes, it's all about being resourceful and cleverly incorporating physical activity into your existing daily routine. Try these workout hacks to maximise your time or to find motivation:

At Home:

- No weights? No problem. Use soup cans, water bottles, or even a bag of rice as weights. The bottom step of your stairs can be a platform for step-ups.

- From YouTube fitness channels to mobile workout apps, there are plenty of resources offering free or inexpensive guided workouts for all fitness levels without even leaving your home.

- Use commercial breaks as mini workout sessions. Do push-ups, sit-ups, squats, or jumping jacks until your show comes back on!

- Sync your workout routine with a friend over a video call. Having someone else to exercise with can provide motivation and accountability.

- Vacuuming, cleaning, gardening—they all burn calories. Try doing them at a faster pace, or incorporate lunges or squats into your routine.

Even the busiest of days can be made healthier with a little creativity and determination!

In the Gym:

- Maximise your gym time by doing exercises that work multiple muscle groups at once, like squats and bench presses.

- High-intensity interval training (HIIT) can give you a full workout in a fraction of the time of a traditional workout.

- Prep your gym bag the night before. This reduces the chances of forgetting something and saves time in the morning. Don't let "not being ready" be an excuse for not going.

- Use the 2-for-1 rule. Instead of resting between sets, do a different exercise that works another part of your body. This keeps your heart rate up and maximises your gym time.

Motivation — Turning Someday, Into Today

Motivation is a key factor when it comes to exercising consistently. Here are some motivation hacks that can help you:

- **Create a playlist:** Music can be a great motivator. Create a workout playlist filled with high-energy songs that make you want to move.

- **Change your perspective:** Instead of viewing exercise as a chore, think of it as "me time" and a chance to de-stress and take care of your body.

- **Reward yourself:** Set up a reward system. For example, treat yourself to a new workout outfit or new pair of trainers after hitting a fitness milestone. Or for every 10 workouts, you could treat yourself to something you've

153

been wanting, like a new book, a massage, or a movie night.

- **Fitness challenges:** Join online fitness challenges. These could be anything from a 30-day yoga challenge to a virtual marathon race. The sense of community can help you stick to your goals, and it's exciting to chart your progress.

- **Fitness Subscription Boxes:** Subscribe to a monthly fitness box that delivers workout gear, healthy snacks, and workout plans to your door. It's a fun surprise that can rekindle your interest in fitness.

- **Exer-gaming:** Video games aren't just for the couch anymore. Many games involve physical activity that can get your heart rate up. Consider investing in a gaming console that encourages movement, such as the Nintendo Switch with games like Ring Fit Adventure— I'm sure there are others.

- **Active social events:** Instead of traditional meet-ups, arrange active social events like hiking, bowling, or a Zumba class with friends. It's a great way to combine fitness and socialising.

- **Charity events:** Sign up for charity runs or walks. The knowledge that you're contributing to a good cause can be a huge motivator. Plus, it's a deadline that can push you to train.

Make exercise a regular part of your routine and if you can do this as part of your everyday life, all the better. The more consistent you are, the more it becomes a habit, and the less motivation you'll need to get to the gym.

Chapter Summary

This chapter served as a toolkit packed with tips to overcome common challenges, tricks to make dieting and workouts easier, and guidance for navigating the nuances of weight loss. These nuggets of wisdom aren't tied to a specific part of the weight loss process but offer valuable insights that will help improve your overall experience. Hopefully, there was something here for you to try. We've covered a lot of ground here, but I don't want you just to pick up one idea and think this alone is the solution. A balanced diet, like the DASH diet, along with regular physical activity is still the cornerstone of any successful weight loss plan.

Chapter 7: DASH Diet Recipes

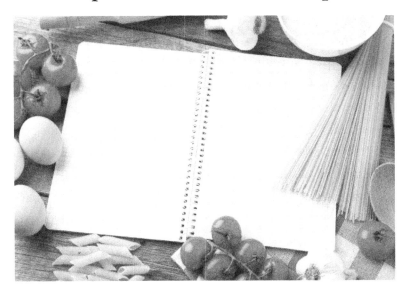

"Healthy eating is a way of life, so it's important to establish routines that are simple, realistically, and ultimately liveable."

—Horace[8]

My favourite part! Here are all of the delicious recipes that have been mentioned throughout the book. Each recipe has been carefully designed to align with the nutritional principles of the DASH diet. These recipes will allow you to confidently experiment in the kitchen while staying true to your health goals. Keep in mind that the recommended daily sodium intake for adults on the DASH diet and the American Heart Association, is no more than 2,300 milligrams (mg) a day, with an ideal limit of no more than 1,500 mg per day for those with

---

[8] Roman lyric poet during the time of Augustus

high blood pressure. These recipes fit well within these guidelines when incorporated into a balanced daily meal plan.

Note that the nutritional values are accurate approximations and are **per serving**. They are estimated, based on the quantities of the specific ingredients listed. The actual nutritional content will vary if you adjust the quantity of ingredients or substitute items. Other factors include the specific brands of canned goods, the seasonings, and other packaged products you use. To help with the measurement conversion, 1 Cup equals 240 grams or 8 fluid ounces. 1 ounce equals 28 grams.

Breakfast

Some people have gotten out of the habit of eating breakfast, relying on lunch to break their fast. If you're not used to eating breakfast, start slowly by adding just a few bites of food to your morning routine. Once you're comfortable with that, gradually increase the amount of food you eat until you're able to eat a full breakfast.

There are many benefits to eating breakfast when trying to lose weight, so stick with it. Breakfast jump starts your metabolism, helping to burn more calories throughout the day. Eating a balanced breakfast also helps to regulate your blood sugar levels, prevent cravings, and overeating later in the day.

Some great options for a healthy weight loss breakfast include oatmeal with fruit, whole grain toast with peanut butter, or cereal with unsweetened almond milk. Whatever you choose, make sure that your breakfast is high in protein and fibre and low in sugar. By following this simple advice, you'll be on your way to starting your day off right and making healthy choices that will help you reach your weight loss goals.

Egg and Vegetable Scramble with Whole Grain Toast

This is the epitome of a nourishing, heart-healthy breakfast. The mix of sautéed vegetables provides a veritable bounty of vitamins and minerals, while the eggs add the high-quality protein.

Serves: 2

Ingredients:

- 4 large eggs
- 1 cup of fresh spinach
- 1/2 bell pepper (diced)
- 1/2 small red onion (diced)
- 1/2 medium tomato (diced)
- 1/2 teaspoon of black pepper)
- 1/2 teaspoon of turmeric
- 2 slices of whole grain bread
- 1 teaspoon of olive oil

Instructions:

1. Heat the olive oil in a non-stick pan over medium heat.
2. Add the bell pepper and onion to the pan. Sauté until tender (5 minutes).
3. Add the spinach and tomatoes, and cook until the spinach wilts.

4. In a bowl, beat the eggs, black pepper, and turmeric. Pour this over the vegetables in the pan.
5. Stir gently on low heat until the eggs are cooked to your liking.
6. Toast the whole grain bread.
7. Serve the scramble with the toasted whole grain bread on the side.

Nutrition: Calories: 255, Protein: 17g, Fat: 13g, Carbs: 19g, Fibre: 4g, Sodium: 218mg

Suggestions: A cup of fresh mixed berries on the side adds a sweet contrast.

Homemade Nutty Granola

When served with low-fat Greek yogurt and fresh and juicy berries, you create a symphony of flavours and textures that make breakfast feel like a treat. Healthy, delicious, and satisfying.

Serves: 10-12
Ingredients:

- 3 cups of oats
- 1 cup of raw almonds (roughly chopped)
- 1/2 cup of raw walnuts (roughly chopped)
- 1/2 cup of raw sunflower seeds
- 1/2 cup of raw pumpkin seeds
- 1/2 cup of unsweetened coconut flakes
- 1/4 cup of flaxseeds
- 1/4 cup of chia seeds

- 1/4 cup of raw honey or pure maple syrup
- 1/4 cup of coconut oil
- 1 teaspoon of pure vanilla extract
- 1-2 teaspoons of cinnamon
- 1 cup of mixed dried fruit (like cranberries, cherries, or chopped apricots)

Instructions:

1. Preheat the oven to 300°F (150°C) and line a baking sheet with parchment paper.
2. In a large bowl, combine the oats, nuts, seeds, and coconut flakes.
3. In a small saucepan, gently and slowly heat the honey, coconut oil, vanilla and cinnamon until well combined.
4. Pour the liquid mixture over the dry ingredients and stir well to coat.
5. Spread the mixture evenly on the baking sheet and bake for 30-40 minutes, stirring every 10 minutes until golden brown.
6. Remove from the oven, and let the mixture cool down. The granola will get crunchier as it cools.
7. Stir in the dried fruit. Store in an airtight container.

Nutrition: Calories: 376, Protein: 9g, Fat: 24g, Carbs: 31g, Fibre: 9g, Sodium: 7mg

Suggestions: Greek yogurt adds a protein boost, and the tartness of the berries perfectly complements the nutty crunch of the granola. This also makes for a great snack at work.

Almond Milk Oatmeal with Cinnamon and Fresh Fruit

This is a hearty, low-fat breakfast that feels indulgent while keeping your health and weight loss goals on track.

Serves: 2

Ingredients:

- 1 cup of oats
- 2 cups of unsweetened almond milk
- 1-2 teaspoons of cinnamon
- 1 cup of mixed fresh fruit (such as blueberries, strawberries and banana slices)

Instructions:

1. In a pot, bring the almond milk to a boil.
2. Add the oats and reduce the heat to low. Allow to simmer, stirring occasionally until the oats are your desired level of tenderness.
3. Stir in the cinnamon.
4. Serve the oatmeal in bowls, topped with the fresh fruit.

Nutrition: Calories: 228, Protein: 7g, Fat: 6g, Carbs: 38g, Fibre: 7g, Sodium: 188mg

Suggestions: Serve with a small glass of apple juice and a handful of raw almonds.

Raspberry Rosewater Overnight Oats

The heart-healthy rolled oats are infused with aromatic rosewater, offering a floral note that pairs wonderfully with the tartness of fresh raspberries. A delicious testament to the potential of the DASH diet!

Serves: 2

Ingredients:

- 1 cup of rolled oats
- 1.5 cups of unsweetened almond milk
- 1/2 cup of fresh raspberries
- 2 tablespoons of chia seeds
- 1 tablespoon of honey or maple syrup (optional)
- 1 teaspoon of rosewater
- 1/4 cup of low-fat Greek yogurt
- Additional raspberries and a sprinkle of unsweetened coconut flakes for a topping

Instructions:

1. In a large bowl, combine the rolled oats, almond milk, raspberries, chia seeds, honey (or maple syrup), and the rosewater. Stir well to combine.
2. Divide the mixture between two mason jars or containers with airtight lids. Cover and refrigerate overnight.
3. In the morning, stir the oats well. They should be thick and creamy. If the mixture is too thick, you can add a little more almond milk.

4. Top each serving with a dollop of Greek yogurt, a few fresh raspberries, and a sprinkle of unsweetened coconut flakes.

Nutrition: Calories: 261, Protein: 8g, Fat: 6g, Carbs 45g, Fibre: 7g, Sodium: 155mg

Suggestions: A piece of whole fruit like a banana or pear for some extra fibre works well if you are gearing up for a full day.

Quinoa Porridge with Fresh Berries and Almonds

This porridge is created by simmering quinoa in almond milk until it attains a creamy consistency. It is similar to traditional oatmeal but with a delicate nutty flavour.

Serves: 2

Ingredients:

- 1 cup of quinoa
- 2 cups of unsweetened almond milk
- 1 cup of mixed fresh berries (such as blueberries, raspberries and blackberries)
- 2 tablespoons of honey (optional)
- A handful of almonds (roughly chopped)

Instructions:

1. Rinse the quinoa under cold water until the water runs clear.
2. In a saucepan, bring water to a boil, then add the quinoa. Reduce the heat to low, cover, and let it simmer

for about 15 minutes, or until the quinoa is tender and the water has been absorbed.

3. Once cooked, remove from the heat and let it stand for 5 minutes. Fluff with a fork.

4. Sweeten the quinoa porridge with honey if desired, and divide it into two bowls.

5. Top each bowl with a mix of fresh berries and a sprinkle of chopped almonds.

Nutrition: Calories: 291, Protein: 8g, Fat: 11g, Carbs: 42g Fibre: 7g, Sodium: 186mg

Suggestions: A cup of green tea or a glass of freshly squeezed grapefruit juice works well.

Chai Spiced Whole Grain Pancakes with Fresh Fruit

These tasty pancakes make a delightfully wholesome and filling breakfast, subtly sweetened with natural honey and applesauce. Delicious!

Serves: 4 (makes about 8 pancakes)

Ingredients:

- 1 cup of whole wheat flour
- 1 cup of rolled oats
- 1 teaspoon of baking powder
- 1/4 teaspoon of ground cinnamon
- 1/4 teaspoon of ground cardamom
- 1/4 teaspoon of ground ginger
- 1/4 teaspoon of ground cloves
- 1/4 teaspoon of ground nutmeg

- 2 tablespoons of unsweetened applesauce
- 1 tablespoon of honey
- 1 egg
- 1.5 cups of unsweetened almond milk
- Fresh mixed berries (strawberries, blueberries and raspberries) for the topping

Instructions:

1. In a large bowl, combine the whole wheat flour, rolled oats, baking powder, and the spices. Mix well.
2. In a separate bowl, whisk together the unsweetened applesauce, honey, egg, and the almond milk.
3. Gradually add the wet ingredients to the dry ingredients, stirring just until combined.
4. Heat a non-stick pan over medium heat. Use a 1/4 cup measure to scoop the batter onto the pan. Cook until bubbles form on the surface, then flip and cook until golden brown.
5. Serve the pancakes topped with fresh mixed berries.

Nutrition: Calories: 245, Protein: 8g, Fat: 4g, Carbs: 44g, Fibre: 4g, Sodium: 90mg

Suggestions: Serve with a small serving of low-fat Greek yogurt. A small glass of freshly squeezed orange juice makes a nice accompaniment.

Whole Grain Toast with Avocado and Boiled Egg

Treat your taste buds to a delightful combination of crunchy, creamy, and savoury with this simple breakfast. This meal is packed with heart-healthy monounsaturated fats from the avocado, and protein from the egg, all layered atop a slice of fibre-rich whole grain bread.

Serves: 2

Ingredients:

- 2 slices of whole grain bread (whole grain rye works well)
- 1 ripe avocado
- 2 large eggs
- Black pepper (optional)

Instructions:

1. This is not a book on how to boil eggs, but this is the way I do it: place the eggs in a saucepan and cover with **cold** water. Bring to a boil over medium-high heat. Once boiling, remove from heat, cover, and let stand for 10 minutes. Remove the eggs from the water, cool, and peel. Perfect eggs!
2. While the eggs are cooking, toast the bread.
3. Cut the avocado in half, remove the stone, and scoop the flesh into a bowl. Mash it lightly with a fork.
4. Spread the mashed avocado evenly onto the toasted bread slices.
5. Slice the boiled eggs and place them on top of the avocado spread. Sprinkle with black pepper if desired.

Nutrition: Calories: 397, Protein: 13g, Fat: 26g, Carbs: 32g, Fibre: 10g, Sodium: 296mg

Suggestions: A small salad of mixed greens and a cup of unsweetened green tea.

Lunch/Dinner

Lunch and dinner are crucial meals where you can incorporate the principles of the DASH diet to its fullest. Emphasise fruits, vegetables, and whole grains: aim to include at least one serving of vegetables in your lunch and two in your dinner. Whole grains should also play a part in your meals; they could be in the form of quinoa, brown rice, or whole grain bread. Choose lean proteins like chicken, fish, lean cuts of meat, or plant-based proteins like lentils and beans. Instead of using salt, try enhancing the flavour of your meals with herbs, spices, or citrus with lemon or lime juice.

As mentioned in chapter 1, planning your meals ahead of time is a game-changer. It reduces the chances of resorting to unhealthy options when you're hungry and short on time. The DASH diet is all about making smart, sustainable choices that contribute to your long-term health, and meal planning is a big part of this.

Baked Chicken Breast with Quinoa Salad and Pomegranate Seeds

The chicken pairs perfectly with the fresh, tangy salad. A feast for the senses with its array of colours, textures, and flavours!

Serves: 4

Ingredients:

- 4 skinless, boneless chicken breasts
- 1 cup of cooked quinoa
- 1 cup of cherry tomatoes (halved)
- 1 cucumber (diced)
- 1 red onion (thinly sliced)
- 1/4 cup of fresh mint (chopped)
- 2 tablespoons of olive oil
- Juice of 1 lemon
- Pepper to taste
- 1 fresh pomegranate

Instructions:

1. Preheat your oven to 375°F (190°C).
2. Season the chicken breasts with pepper, and a drizzle of olive oil. Place them in a baking dish and bake for about 20-25 minutes, or until they're cooked through.
3. While the chicken is baking, prepare the quinoa salad. In a large bowl, combine the cooked quinoa, cherry tomatoes, cucumber, red onion, and the mint.
4. Cut the pomegranate in half and remove the seeds. Add these to the salad.
5. Dress the salad with olive oil, lemon juice, pepper, and mix everything together.
6. Once the chicken is done, let it rest for a few minutes before slicing.
7. Serve each chicken breast with a generous serving of the quinoa salad.

Nutrition: Calories: 400, Protein: 30g, Fat: 14g, Carbs: 35g, Fibre: 6g, Sodium: 300mg

Suggestions: This meal pairs nicely with a side of steamed asparagus drizzled with a squeeze of fresh lemon juice.

Baked Salmon with Lemon and Dill

Perfect for a weeknight meal, yet elegant enough for a dinner party. This dish is a testament to the magic that can happen when a few simple, high-quality ingredients, are prepared with care.

Serves: 4

Ingredients:

- 4 salmon fillets (about 4-6 ounces each)
- 1 lemon, thinly sliced
- 4 sprigs of fresh dill
- Pepper to taste
- 1 tablespoon of olive oil

Instructions:

1. Preheat your oven to 400°F (200°C).
2. Place the salmon fillets on a baking sheet lined with parchment paper. Season each fillet with the pepper, then top with lemon slices and a sprig of dill.
3. Drizzle the olive oil over the salmon fillets.
4. Bake for about 15 minutes, or until the salmon is cooked through and flakes easily with a fork.

Nutrition: Calories: 350, Protein: 34g, Fat: 23g, Carbs: 1g, Fibre: 1g, Sodium: 250 mg

Suggestions: For an accompanying side dish, consider a serving of quinoa, cherry tomatoes and cucumbers, or steamed asparagus with a squeeze of lemon.

Chickpea and Vegetable Curry

A comforting meal that's bursting with flavour and packed with nutrition. The chickpeas provide a healthy dose of fibre and plant-based protein, while the vegetables provide a variety of essential nutrients.

Serves: 6

Ingredients:

- 2 cans of chickpeas (drained and rinsed)
- 1 tablespoon of olive oil
- 1 medium onion (diced)
- 2 cloves garlic (minced)
- 1 tablespoon of fresh ginger (grated)
- 1 medium red bell pepper (diced)
- 1 medium zucchini (diced)
- 2 teaspoons of curry powder
- 1 teaspoon of turmeric
- 1 can of tomatoes
- 1 can of light coconut milk
- Pepper to taste
- Fresh cilantro for garnish

Instructions:

1. In a large pan, heat the olive oil over a medium heat.

2. Add the onion, garlic, and ginger, and cook until the onion is translucent.
3. Stir in the curry powder and the turmeric. Add the bell pepper and zucchini.
4. Add the chickpeas, the diced tomatoes (with the juice), and the coconut milk.
5. Bring the mixture to a simmer, then reduce the heat to low, cover, and let it cook for about 30-40 minutes. Stir occasionally.
6. Season with pepper to taste, and garnish with fresh cilantro before serving.

Nutrition: Calories: 275, Protein: 10g, Fat: 10g, Carbs: 35g, Fibre: 10g, Sodium 350mg

Suggestions: For an accompanying side dish, a serving of brown basmati rice or a warm whole grain naan bread works well.

Chilli Non Carne and Cauliflower Rice

Chilli Non Carne and Cauliflower Rice is a warm, hearty, and flavour-packed dish that will satisfy your cravings while keeping you on track with the DASH diet. This meal is a wonderful example of how low-fat, low-sodium foods can be delicious, satisfying, and aid in weight loss.

Serves: 4

Ingredients:

- 1 large cauliflower
- 2 tablespoons of olive oil
- 1 large onion (diced)

- 2 garlic cloves (minced)
- 1 red bell pepper (diced)
- 1 can of black beans (rinsed and drained)
- 1 can of kidney beans (rinsed and drained)
- 1 can of diced tomatoes (no salt added)
- 1 teaspoon of chilli powder
- 1 teaspoon of cumin
- Black pepper to taste

Instructions:

1. Cut the cauliflower into florets, removing the stems. Pulse in a food processor until they reach a rice-like consistency. You can also do this by hand with a large knife.
2. In a large pan, heat 1 tablespoon of the olive oil. Add the cauliflower rice, stirring occasionally until cooked for around 5 minutes. Set aside.
3. In the same pan, add the remaining oil, onion, garlic, and the diced red bell pepper. Sauté until soft.
4. Add the beans, tomatoes, chilli powder, cumin, and black pepper. Simmer for about 15-20 minutes, stirring occasionally.

Nutrition: Calories: 340, Protein: 14g, Fat: 8g, Carbs: 52g, Fibre: 16g, Sodium: 120mg

Suggestions: Serve with a crisp green salad with an apple cider vinegar and lemon dressing.

Greek Salad with Grilled Chicken and Roasted Chickpeas

The lean chicken and crispy roasted chickpeas add a protein punch to this salad, while the vegetables bring a medley of refreshing textures and flavours.

Serves: 4

Ingredients:

- 2 boneless, skinless chicken breasts
- 1 tablespoon of olive oil
- Black pepper to taste
- 1 head of romaine lettuce (chopped)
- 1 cucumber (sliced)
- 2 tomatoes (diced)
- 1 red onion (thinly sliced)
- 1/4 cup of pitted Kalamata olives
- 1/2 cup of low sodium feta cheese (crumbled)
- 1 can of chickpeas, rinsed, drained, and patted dry
- 1 teaspoon of smoked paprika
- Juice of 1 lemon

Instructions:

1. Preheat the grill to a medium heat. Brush the chicken breasts with olive oil and season with black pepper. Grill until cooked through (8-10 minutes per side). Let them rest for a few minutes, then slice.
2. Meanwhile, preheat the oven to 400°F (200°C). Toss the chickpeas in the olive oil and smoked paprika.

Spread on a baking sheet and roast for about 20 minutes, or until crispy.

3. In a large bowl, combine all the ingredients. Drizzle with lemon juice.

Nutrition: Calories: 350, Protein: 30g, Fat: 12g, Carbs: 28g, Fibre: 8g, Sodium: 300mg

Suggestions: Serve with a warmed whole grain pita bread, toasted and cut into wedges. I find that just popping into a toaster for 2 minutes or so works well!

Grilled Chicken Salad with Mixed Greens and Avocado Dressing

A vibrant mix of juicy grilled chicken, fresh vegetables, and sweet pomegranate seeds, all tied together with a creamy, tangy avocado dressing. This will satisfy your hunger while keeping your health goals in check.

Serves: 4

Ingredients:

- 4 boneless, skinless chicken breasts
- 8 cups of mixed salad greens
- 2 cups cherry tomatoes (halved)
- 1 cucumber (sliced)
- 1 ripe avocado
- 2 tablespoons of fresh lemon juice
- 1 tablespoon of olive oil
- 1/2 cup of unsweetened almond milk
- Pepper to taste
- 1 cup of pomegranate seeds

Instructions:

1. Season the chicken breasts with pepper, then grill on a medium heat for about 8-10 minutes per side until no longer pink in the centre. Allow to cool, then slice.
2. In a blender, combine the ripe avocado, lemon juice, olive oil, almond milk and pepper. Blend until smooth to create the avocado dressing.
3. In a large bowl, mix the salad greens, cherry tomatoes, cucumber, and the sliced chicken.
4. Drizzle the avocado dressing over the salad and gently mix to combine.
5. Top the salad with pomegranate seeds before serving.

Nutrition: Calories: 300, Protein: 25g, Fat: 15g, Carbs: 15g, Fibre: 7g, Sodium: 140mg

Suggestions: Serve this salad alongside a hearty whole grain roll for added fibre.

Grilled Chicken Wrap with Raspberry Chipotle Sauce

A vibrant, flavourful twist on a lunch classic. The unusual star of the show, the raspberry chipotle sauce, adds a delightful combination of sweetness, smokiness, and a touch of heat to the wrap—elevating the wrap from the ordinary to the extraordinary!

Serves: 4

Ingredients:

- 2 boneless, skinless chicken breasts
- 1 tablespoon of olive oil
- Black pepper to taste
- 4 whole wheat tortillas
- 2 cups of mixed greens
- 1/2 cup of cherry tomatoes (halved)
- 1/2 a red onion (thinly sliced)
- 1/2 cup of grated carrot
- 1/2 cup of fresh raspberries
- 1 teaspoon of hot chipotle pepper puree/paste (look for reduced sodium)
- 1 tablespoon of apple cider vinegar

Instructions:

1. Preheat the grill to a medium heat. Brush the chicken breasts with olive oil and season with black pepper. Grill until cooked through, about 8-10 minutes per side. Let them rest for a few minutes, then slice.
2. For the sauce, blend the raspberries, chipotle pepper, and apple cider vinegar until smooth.
3. Warm the tortillas on a dry frying pan over medium heat (or microwave for 20 seconds).
4. Divide the mixed greens, cherry tomatoes, red onion, and grated carrot among the tortillas. Add the grilled chicken and drizzle with the raspberry chipotle sauce. Roll up the tortillas and get ready for a taste extravaganza!

Nutrition: Calories: 290, Protein: 25g, Fat: 7g, Carbs: 33g, Fibre: 5g, Sodium: 220mg

Suggestions: Freshly juiced apple; eating these is thirsty work!

Grilled Fish with Pomegranate Salsa, Roasted Brussels Sprouts and Sweet Potatoes

A low-fat, low-sodium feast for your taste buds that will leave you nourished and satiated.

Serves: 4

Ingredients:

- 4 white fish fillets (like cod or halibut)
- 1 tablespoon of olive oil
- Black pepper to taste
- 1 cup of pomegranate seeds
- 1/2 cup of diced cucumber
- 1/2 cup of chopped fresh cilantro
- 1 lime (juiced)
- 2 cups of Brussels sprouts (halved)
- 2 sweet potatoes (cubed)
- 1 tablespoon of ground cinnamon

Instructions:

1. Preheat the grill to a medium heat. Brush the fish fillets with olive oil and season with black pepper. Grill until the fish flakes easily with a fork (about 5 minutes per side).

2. In a bowl, mix the pomegranate seeds, diced cucumber, chopped cilantro, and lime juice to create the salsa. Set aside.

3. Preheat the oven to 400°F (200°C). Toss the Brussels sprouts and sweet potatoes with 1 tablespoon of olive oil and sprinkle with cinnamon. Roast until golden and tender (20-25 minutes).

Nutrition: Calories: 325, Protein: 30g, Fat: 8g, Carbs: 35g, Fibre: 8g, Sodium: 150mg

Suggestions: A crisp green salad with an oil-free lemon vinaigrette.

Greek Yoghurt Chicken

Greek yoghurt chicken is the perfect combination of health and flavour. The simplicity of the dish brings out the clean, delicious flavours. It's a meal you'll look forward to again and again.

Serves: 4

Ingredients:

- 4 boneless, skinless chicken breasts
- 1 cup Greek yoghurt
- 2 cloves of garlic (minced)
- 1 tablespoon of lemon juice
- 1 tablespoon fresh dill, chopped (or 1 teaspoon of dried dill)
- Pepper to taste

Instructions:

1. In a bowl, combine the Greek yoghurt, minced garlic, lemon juice, dill and the pepper. Mix until well combined.
2. Add the chicken breasts to the yoghurt mixture, making sure each piece is thoroughly coated. Let the chicken marinate for at least an hour in the refrigerator, or ideally, overnight.
3. Preheat your oven to 375°F (190°C) and line a baking dish with foil or parchment paper.
4. Arrange the marinated chicken breasts in the prepared baking dish. Bake for around 30 minutes, or until the chicken is cooked through and no longer pink in the middle.
5. Let the chicken rest for a few minutes before serving,

Nutrition: Calories: 180, Protein: 28g, Fat: 4g, Carbs: 3g, Fibre: 0g, Sodium 350 mg

Suggestions: Serve with a side of steamed vegetables, or a fresh salad for a complete meal.

Quinoa Salad with Roasted Vegetables

Ideal as a stand-alone lunch or as a side with your choice of lean protein for dinner. This is a versatile dish that you will love having in your DASH diet repertoire. Heart-healthy, packed with fibre, and low in sodium, making it perfect for those keeping a close watch on their salt intake.

Serves: 4

Ingredients:

- 1 cup uncooked quinoa
- 2 cups vegetable stock/broth (look for low sodium if store bought)
- 3 cups mixed vegetables (e.g., bell peppers, zucchini, carrots, red onion)
- 1 tablespoon olive oil
- Pepper to taste

For the dressing:

- 1 tablespoon light olive oil
- 1 tablespoon lemon juice
- 1 garlic clove (minced)
- Pepper to taste

Instructions:

1. Preheat your oven to 400°F (200°C).
2. Toss the mixed vegetables in olive oil and pepper. Spread them out on a baking sheet and roast for about 20-25 minutes, or until tender and lightly browned.
3. While the vegetables are roasting, rinse the quinoa under cold water until the water runs clear. Combine the quinoa and the vegetable stock in a saucepan. Bring to a boil, then reduce the heat. Cover and let it simmer for about 15 minutes or until the quinoa is tender and the stock is absorbed.
4. To make the dressing, whisk together the olive oil, lemon juice, minced garlic and pepper.

5. Fluff the quinoa with a fork and let it cool slightly. Combine the quinoa, roasted vegetables, and dressing in a large bowl. Mix until everything is evenly coated in the dressing.

6. You can serve this salad warm or chilled.

Nutrition: Calories: 253, Protein: 7g, Fat: 10g, Carbs: 35g, Fibre: 6g, Sodium: 89 mg

Suggestions: This salad is flexible, so feel free to add other ingredients you like, such as roasted nuts and dried fruit. Green beans work well.

Shrimp Stir-Fry with Mixed Vegetables and a Serving of Brown Rice

Succulent shrimp, crunchy vegetables, and tropical mango cubes, with a dash of light soy sauce. Served with fluffy brown rice, it offers savoury, sweet, and umami flavours without overloading on sodium. A delight for your tastebuds!

Serves: 4

Ingredients:

- 1 lb of shrimp (peeled and deveined)
- 1 cup of bell peppers (sliced)
- 1 cup of broccoli florets
- 1 cup of sugar snap peas
- 1 cup of carrots (sliced)
- 2 cloves of garlic (minced)
- 2 tablespoons of low sodium soy sauce (this is still relatively high in sodium, so watch your daily totals)

- 1 tablespoon of olive oil
- Pepper to taste
- 2 cups of cooked brown rice
- 1 fresh mango, peeled and cubed

Instructions:

1. Heat the olive oil in a large pan over medium heat. Add the garlic and saute until fragrant.
2. Add the shrimp to the pan and cook until they're pink, about 4-5 minutes. Remove the shrimp and set them aside.
3. In the same pan, add the bell peppers, broccoli, sugar snap peas, and the carrots. Sauté until they're tender (about 5 minutes).
4. Return the shrimp to the pan, add the soy sauce, and stir well to combine. Season with pepper to taste.
5. Stir in the fresh mango cubes, and cook for an additional minute.
6. Serve the shrimp stir-fry over a bed of brown rice.

Nutrition: Calories: 388, Protein: 32g, Fat: 9g, Carbs: 50g, Fibre: 7g, Sodium: 442mg

Suggestions: This shrimp stir-fry pairs perfectly with a simple Asian-inspired cucumber salad for a refreshing crunch.

Spicy Shrimp and Avocado Lettuce Wraps

Combined with a tangy burst from the lime, and you've got a wrap that's truly an explosion of flavours in every bite. Light, yet satisfying. Delicious and healthy at the same time.

Serves: 4

Ingredients:

- 1 lb of shrimp, peeled and deveined
- 1 tablespoon olive oil
- 1/2 teaspoon cayenne pepper
- Pepper to taste
- 1 ripe avocado (sliced)
- 1 medium tomato, (diced)
- 1 small red onion (finely chopped)
- Juice of 1 lime
- 8-10 large lettuce leaves (romaine or iceberg)

Instructions:

1. Heat the olive oil in a pan over a medium heat. Add the shrimp and cayenne pepper. Sauté until the shrimp are cooked through and pink, about 4-5 minutes.
2. In a separate bowl, combine the diced avocado, tomato, and red onion. Squeeze in the lime juice and add a pinch of pepper, then stir to combine.
3. To assemble the wraps, place a scoop of the avocado mixture onto each lettuce leaf, then top with the cooked shrimp.
4. Serve the wraps immediately!

Nutrition: Calories: 286, Protein: 27g, Fat: 15g, Carbs: 10g, Fibre: 5g, Sodium 282mg

Suggestions: Accompany these delicious wraps with a side of fresh fruit salad for a light, refreshing finish to your meal.

Spinach and Low-Sodium Feta Stuffed Chicken Breast

This stuffed chicken breast is not only delectable but also packed with protein. A gourmet-style meal that you can make at home that is sure to impress your tastebuds and your friends!

Serves: 4

Ingredients:

- 4 boneless, skinless chicken breasts
- 2 cups of fresh spinach (chopped)
- 1/2 cup low-sodium feta cheese (crumbled)
- 2 cloves of garlic (minced)
- 1 tablespoon of olive oil
- Pepper to taste

Instructions:

1. Preheat your oven to 375°F (190°C).
2. Cut a pocket into the side of each chicken breast. Be careful not to cut all the way through.
3. In a frying pan, heat the olive oil over medium heat. Add the garlic and cook until fragrant.
4. Add the spinach and cook until just wilted.
5. Remove the frying pan from the heat and stir in the feta cheese.

6. Stuff each chicken breast with the spinach and feta mixture. You can seal and secure these with toothpicks if needed.

7. Season the chicken with pepper and place on a baking sheet lined with parchment paper.

8. Bake for about 30 minutes, or until the chicken is cooked through and no longer pink in the middle.

Nutrition: Calories: 300 Protein: 28g, Fat: 20g, Carbs: 3g, Fibre: 1g, Sodium 320mg

Suggestions: For an accompanying side dish, consider roasted baby potatoes tossed in rosemary and a squeeze of lemon. Or keep it simple with a fresh mixed green salad with a balsamic vinaigrette.

Sweet Potato and Black Bean Tacos

A vibrant and satisfying dish that combines hearty, sweet roasted sweet potatoes, creamy avocado, and protein-rich black beans, all served inside a soft corn tortilla. Nutritious, packed with fibre, and bursting with colour and flavour.

Serves: 4 (2 tacos per serving)

Ingredients:

- 2 medium sweet potatoes (peeled and diced)
- 1 tablespoon of olive oil
- 1 teaspoon of chilli powder
- Pepper to taste
- 1 can of black beans (drained and rinsed)
- 8 small corn tortillas

- 1 ripe avocado (diced)
- Fresh cilantro and lime wedges for serving

Instructions:

1. Preheat your oven to 400°F (200°C). Toss the diced sweet potatoes in olive oil, chilli powder and pepper, then spread them out on a baking sheet. Roast for about 20 minutes, or until tender and lightly browned.
2. Warm the black beans in a small pot over a low heat.
3. To assemble the tacos, spread a spoonful of warm black beans on each tortilla, then top with the roasted sweet potatoes and diced avocado.
4. Serve the tacos garnished with fresh cilantro and a squeeze of lime juice.

Nutrition: Calories: 354, Protein: 10g, Fat: 15g, Carbs: 49g, Fibre: 13g, Sodium 61mg

Suggestions: For an accompanying side dish, consider a refreshing salad or a serving of brown rice.

Turkey and Quinoa Stuffed Bell Peppers

Topped with a layer of melted low-fat cheddar cheese, these stuffed peppers are a satisfying meal in itself. High in protein and fibre, yet low in fat. It's comfort food you can feel good about!

Serves: 4

Ingredients:

- 4 large bell peppers (tops cut off and seeds removed)
- 1 lb of lean ground turkey
- 1 cup of cooked quinoa
- 1 small onion (finely chopped)
- 2 cloves garlic (minced)
- 1 can of diced tomatoes (drained)
- 1 teaspoon of ground cumin
- 1 teaspoon of chilli powder
- Pepper to taste
- 1/2 cup grated low-fat cheddar cheese (low sodium)

Instructions:

1. Preheat your oven to 375°F (190°C).
2. In a large frying pan, cook the ground turkey, onion, and the garlic over a medium heat until the turkey is no longer pink.
3. Stir in the quinoa, diced tomatoes, cumin, chilli powder and the pepper.
4. With a spoon, fill each bell pepper with the turkey and quinoa stuffing mixture, then place them in a baking dish.
5. Cover with foil and bake for 20 minutes.
6. Remove the foil, sprinkle the cheese on top of each pepper, and bake for another 10 or so, until the cheese is melted and bubbly.

Nutrition: Calories: 404, Protein: 33g, Fat: 15g, Carbs: 36g, Fibre: 6g, Sodium 199mg

Suggestions: For an accompanying side dish, consider a simple mixed greens salad with a light vinaigrette or steamed broccoli with a squeeze of lemon.

Turkey Meatballs with Marinara Sauce over Spaghetti Squash

A twist on a classic, offering robust flavours with a lighter, healthier touch. Perfect for those seeking comfort with a DASH of nutrition.

Serves: 4

Ingredients:

- 1 large spaghetti squash
- 1 lb of ground turkey
- 1 large egg
- 1/4 cup of whole wheat bread crumbs
- Black pepper to taste
- 2 cups of low-sodium marinara sauce
- Fresh basil leaves for garnish

Instructions:

1. Preheat the oven to 400°F (200°C). Slice the spaghetti squash in half lengthwise, scoop out the seeds. Place cut side down on a baking sheet. Roast for 40-50 minutes or until the flesh is tender and shreds easily with a fork.
2. Meanwhile, in a bowl, combine the ground turkey, egg, bread crumbs, and the black pepper. Form into evenly sized meatballs.

189

3. Bake the meatballs on a separate baking sheet in the preheated oven for 20-25 minutes, or until cooked through and browned on the outside.

4. In a saucepan, heat the marinara sauce over medium heat and simmer for 10 minutes.

5. Serve the cooked meatballs and marinara sauce over the spaghetti squash. Garnish with fresh basil leaves.

Nutrition: Calories: 380, Protein: 35g, Fat: 10g, Carbs: 45g, Fibre: 6g, Sodium: 140mg

Suggestions: A colourful salad of mixed greens, cherry tomatoes, cucumber and a splash of balsamic vinegar.

Vegetable Stir-fry with Tofu

The tofu, lightly crisped and golden, is a perfect protein-packed base for the stir-fried vegetables. Fresh garlic and ginger add a warm aromatic backbone to the dish.

Serves: 4

Ingredients:

- 14 ounces firm tofu (drained and cubed)
- 1 tablespoon of sesame oil
- 1 red bell pepper (thinly sliced)
- 1 yellow bell pepper (thinly sliced)
- 2 medium carrots (sliced into thin rounds)
- 2 cloves of garlic (minced)
- 2 teaspoons of freshly grated ginger
- 1 tablespoon of low-sodium soy sauce or tamari (light)
- 1 tablespoon of rice vinegar

- 2 green onions (sliced)
- Sesame seeds for garnish

Instructions:

1. Heat half the sesame oil in a wok or large frying pan over a medium heat. Add the tofu and cook until golden on all sides. Remove from the pan and set aside.
2. Add the remaining sesame oil to the pan, then add the peppers, carrots, garlic, and ginger. Stir-fry for around 5 minutes, or until the vegetables are just tender.
3. Return the tofu to the pan, add the soy sauce and rice vinegar, and stir well. Cook for another 2 minutes to allow the flavours to blend.
4. Serve the stir-fry garnished with sliced green onions and sesame seeds.

Nutrition: Calories: 144, Protein: 10g, Fat: 8g, Carbs: 11g, Fibre: 3g, Sodium 186mg

Suggestions: For an accompanying side dish, consider a bowl of steamed brown rice or a light cucumber salad.

Zucchini Zoodle Noodles with Pesto and Cherry Tomatoes

The zucchini noodles, or zoodles, are a fun and low-carb substitute for traditional pasta. Their mild flavour works well with the rich pesto.

Serves: 4

Ingredients:

- 4 medium zucchinis
- 1 cup of fresh basil leaves
- 1/4 cup of pine nuts
- 2 cloves of garlic
- 1/4 cup of extra virgin olive oil
- 1/2 cup of grated Parmesan cheese
- Pepper to taste
- 1 cup cherry tomatoes (halved)

Instructions:

1. Using a spiraliser, make noodles out of the zucchinis.
2. In a food processor, combine the basil leaves, pine nuts, and garlic. Slowly add the olive oil while the food processor is running. Once smooth, add the Parmesan cheese and season with the pepper.
3. Toss the zucchini noodles with the pesto. Top with cherry tomatoes and serve.

Nutrition: Calories: 321, Protein: 16g, Fat: 26g, Carbs: 11g, Fibre: 4g, Sodium: 340mg

Suggestions: For an accompanying side dish, consider a simple arugula (rocket) salad with lemon vinaigrette, or a slice of whole grain garlic bread—go easy on the butter!

Bonus Recipe: DASH Diet No-Crust Pizza!

By popular demand, here is a bonus for you—No-crust pizza! This recipe substitutes traditional crust with portobello mushrooms, delivering all the pizza flavour you love with a fraction of the sodium and calories.

Serves: 4

Ingredients:

- 4 large portobello mushroom caps (the larger the better)
- 1 cup of low-sodium marinara sauce
- 1 cup of shredded part-skim mozzarella cheese (low sodium)
- 1 bell pepper (thinly sliced)
- 1/2 red onion (thinly sliced)
- 2 cups of fresh spinach
- 1/2 teaspoon of dried oregano
- 1/2 teaspoon of dried basil
- Freshly ground black pepper to taste
- Olive oil spray

Instructions:

1. Preheat your oven to 375°F (190°C). Line a baking sheet with parchment paper.
2. Clean the portobello caps and remove the stems. Spray the underside of the mushrooms with olive oil and place them on the prepared baking sheet.
3. Spread a quarter of the marinara sauce on each mushroom cap. Then distribute the shredded mozzarella evenly over the sauce.

4. Arrange the sliced bell peppers, red onion, and spinach evenly over the cheese.

5. Sprinkle the pizzas with oregano, basil, and freshly ground black pepper.

6. Bake for 15 minutes or until the cheese is melted and bubbly.

7. Let the pizzas cool for a few minutes before serving.

8. Enjoy your heart-healthy, DASH diet-friendly, no-crust pizza!

Nutrition: Calories: 185, Protein: 16g, Fat: 10g, Carbs: 10g, Fibre: 2g, Sodium: 390mg

Suggestions: Serve with a crisp green salad and an apple cider vinegar and lemon dressing.

Snacks and Dips

As with all these dips, freshly chopped raw vegetables like bell peppers, cucumber, carrot, celery, cherry tomatoes, and whole grain pita bread are all ideal for dipping.

Homemade Low-Fat Baba Ghanoush

This creamy dip is bursting with the smoky flavour of roasted eggplant, combined with the nuttiness of the tahini and a zesty kick from the fresh lemon juice. Garlic and cumin add depth to the overall flavour. Perfect for a healthy snack, appetiser, or light lunch!

Serves: 6

Ingredients:

- 2 medium eggplants
- 2 cloves of garlic (minced)

- Juice of 1 lemon
- 2 tablespoons of tahini
- 1 tablespoon of olive oil
- 1/2 teaspoon of ground cumin
- 2 tablespoons of fresh parsley (chopped)
- Ground black pepper to taste

Instructions:

1. Preheat your oven to 400°F (200°C). Prick the eggplants all over with a fork and place on a baking sheet.
2. Roast the eggplants in the oven for about 40-45 minutes until they're soft.
3. Let the eggplants cool, then slice them open and scoop out the flesh. Discard the skins.
4. In a food processor, combine the eggplant flesh, garlic, lemon juice, tahini, olive oil, and the cumin. Blend until smooth.
5. Transfer to a serving dish and mix in the fresh parsley. Season with ground black pepper to taste.

Nutrition: Calories: 93, Protein: 3g, Fat: 5g, Carbs: 11g, Fibre: 6g, Sodium: 10mg

Homemade Low-Fat Muhammara

The sweetness of roasted red bell peppers combines with the crunch of walnuts and the warmth of the spices. Perfect as a spread or a dip.

Serves: 6

Ingredients:

- 3 red bell peppers
- 1 cup of walnuts
- 2 cloves of garlic
- Juice of 1 lemon
- 1 teaspoon ground cumin
- 1 teaspoon of paprika
- 1/2 cup of whole grain bread crumbs
- 2 tablespoons of pomegranate molasses
- 2 tablespoons of olive oil

Instructions:

1. Preheat your oven to 400°F (200°C). Place the red bell peppers on a baking sheet and roast in the oven for about 25-30 minutes, or until the skins are completely wrinkly and the peppers are charred.
2. Remove the peppers from the oven and let them cool. Once cooled, remove the skins and seeds.
3. In a food processor, combine the roasted peppers, walnuts, garlic, lemon juice, cumin, paprika, bread crumbs, pomegranate molasses, and olive oil. Blend until smooth.
4. Transfer to a serving dish and garnish with a few chopped walnuts and a drizzle of pomegranate molasses.

Nutrition: Calories: 248, Protein: 7g, Fat: 17g, Carbs: 21g, Fibre: 3g, Sodium: 59mg

Low-Fat, No-Salt Homemade Hummus

Try this low-fat, no-salt hummus as a well-balanced snack or appetiser. A smooth and flavourful dip that satisfies without overloading on fat or salt.

Serves: 8

Ingredients:

- 2 cups canned chickpeas, drained (reserve the liquid)
- 2 cloves of garlic
- 1/3 cup of fresh lemon juice
- 1/2 cup of tahini
- 2 tablespoons of olive oil
- 1/2 teaspoon of ground cumin
- 1/4 teaspoon of paprika
- Fresh parsley for garnish

Instructions:

1. In a food processor, combine the chickpeas, garlic, lemon juice, tahini, olive oil, cumin, and paprika.
2. Blend until smooth. Add the reserved chickpea liquid a little at a time until you reach your desired consistency.
3. Transfer the hummus to a bowl and garnish with a sprinkle of paprika and fresh parsley.

Nutrition: Calories: 306, Protein: 12g, Fat: 15g, Carbs: 34g, Fibre: 10g, Sodium: 32mg

Conclusion

"You didn't gain all your weight in one day; you won't lose it in one day. Be patient with yourself." Jenna Wolfe[9]

As we conclude this book let's remind ourselves that this process is not just about shedding pounds but about fostering a healthier, more vibrant lifestyle. It's about making sustainable changes that lead to long-lasting benefits. Setbacks are a part of any significant lifestyle change. Whether it's a plateau in weight loss, finding it hard to stick to the diet, or skipping a few workouts, the key is to accept these moments as temporary, and keep going. Scientific literature stresses the importance of resilience in weight loss efforts, emphasising that a single setback does not equate to overall failure. Adapt your plans, revisit your goals, and accept that progress is not always linear.

Beyond weight loss, the adoption of the DASH diet and regular exercise can bring numerous health benefits. Improved cardiovascular health, enhanced mood, increased energy levels, and better sleep quality are all there for the taking. This journey is less about reaching a specific weight and more about developing healthy habits that will serve you well for a lifetime.

In the words of Dr. Kenneth H. Cooper, considered the father of the fitness movement, "Fitness is a journey, not a destination." Keep this in mind as you navigate your own path to health. Celebrate every success, no matter how small. Every time you choose a nutrient-rich meal, every time you decide to

---

[9] Journalist and personal trainer

move your body—these are victories. They reflect your commitment to your health and your well-being.

As a scientist, I can provide you with evidence, advice, and recommendations. But as a fellow human, my final words are these: Be patient with yourself. Be proud of your progress. And most importantly, enjoy this journey of self-improvement and self-discovery. It's a journey filled with challenges and victories, lessons and growth, and ultimately, a journey towards a healthier, happier, and more vibrant you.

You've got this!

Glossary of Terms

These terms were used in the book. Understanding these terms will further enhance your knowledge of the DASH diet and contribute to a successful weight loss journey.

Anthocyanins: Anthocyanins are found in a variety of plants and are known for their antioxidant properties and potential health benefits. They are found in the bark and skin of certain fruits like grapes, apples, and berries. They are also present in red wine, chocolate, and certain types of tea.

Carb Creep: This term describes the gradual and often unnoticed increase in carbohydrate consumption. This can occur when following an initial low-carbohydrate diet, or indeed, any diet. Carbs are just too easy to eat and we need to be conscious of this.

Cholecystokinin: Cholecystokinin (CCK) is secreted by cells in the duodenum (the first part of the small intestine). It stimulates the release of digestive enzymes from the pancreas from the gallbladder. Cholecystokinin helps in reducing appetite.

Dopamine: A neurotransmitter, also known as the 'reward chemical'. It plays a role in how we perceive pleasure and reward. It therefore contributes to motivation, drive, and overall mood. The good news is dopamine is released in the brain when we engage in activities that we find enjoyable or rewarding; exercise included!

Empty Calories: This term refers to calories derived from foods (or drinks) that contain little or no nutritional value. These foods or beverages are often high in processed sugars and unhealthy fats but lack beneficial nutrients like vitamins, minerals, fibre, and protein.

Endorphins: Endorphins are a type of neurotransmitter that help relieve pain and stress. Similar to dopamine, they are often referred to as the body's 'feel-good' chemicals because they interact with the opiate receptors in the brain.

Gene Expression: Refers to the process by which the information encoded in a gene is used to direct the assembly of a protein molecule.

Ghrelin: Ghrelin is a hormone produced in the stomach and, to a lesser extent, in the small intestine, pancreas, and brain. It is often referred to as the 'hunger hormone' and it plays a role in regulating appetite and energy homeostasis.

GLP-1: A key hormone involved in digestion and appetite regulation. GLP-1 is secreted by cells in the small intestine and brain in response to food intake.

Glutes: Short for gluteus muscles. The glutes are a group of three muscles that make up the buttocks: the gluteus maximus, gluteus medius, and gluteus minimus.

Glycerol: A compound that plays a role in the body's metabolism. It is the backbone of triglycerides; the main type of fat found in the body.

Glycogen: A type of carbohydrate that is stored in the body's muscles and liver. Glycogen serves as a form of energy storage that can be quickly used when needed.

Hamstrings: The hamstrings refer to the group of three muscles located at the back of the thigh. They play a crucial role in walking, running, and jumping by helping to bend the knee.

HDL (High-Density Lipoprotein): Known as 'good cholesterol'. HDL carries cholesterol from the body's cells back to the liver for disposal or recycling.

Hunger Hormones: Refer to the biochemical substances produced within the body that play a role in regulating hunger and satiety. The two primary hunger hormones are ghrelin and leptin.

Hypertension: High blood pressure. This is a medical condition where the force exerted by the blood against the walls of the arteries is too high. This can lead to harmful health conditions such as heart disease and stroke. Hypertension develops over many years. People with hypertension may not have any noticeable symptoms.

Lactate: A compound produced by the body during intense exercise. Lactate is actually a byproduct of anaerobic metabolism. This happens when there is not enough oxygen to produce energy in the muscles.

LDL (Low-Density Lipoprotein): Referred to as 'bad cholesterol'. LDL carries cholesterol from the liver to cells throughout the body. An excessive amount of LDL can lead to the build-up of cholesterol in the arterial walls.

Leptin: Leptin is produced in fat cells. It sends signals to the brain to suppress hunger and also indicates fullness.

Meta-analysis: A statistical and scientific method used to consolidate the results of several independent studies.

NHLBI: The National Heart, Lung, and Blood Institute (NHLBI) is a component of the U.S. National Institutes of Health (NIH). It holds the responsibility for improving the health of citizens of the United States.

Peptide YY: Peptide YY is produced in the gut after eating. It reduces appetite by acting on neurons in the brain that regulate satiety.

Quads: Short for quadriceps. These are the group of four large muscles located at the front of the thigh. The primary function of the quads is to extend the knee, required for walking, running and jumping.

Refined Carbs: This term refers to carbohydrates that have been processed and stripped of their natural nutrients and fibre. Examples of refined carbs include white flour, white rice, and sugars. These are often used in processed foods.

Serotonin: A neurotransmitter that plays a role in mood regulation, appetite, sleep, memory, and learning. Higher levels of serotonin generally lead to feelings of happiness and well-being.

Systematic Review: Refers to a rigorous and comprehensive literature review that involves a detailed and scientific search for relevant studies on a specific topic.

Triglycerides: Lipid (fat) molecules found in the bloodstream. They serve as a main form of energy storage in the body. High levels of triglycerides in the blood can be an indicator of an increased risk of heart disease.

Julia E. Chatwin

Thank You

Thank you for choosing to spend your valuable time exploring DASH, exercise, and weight loss with me. I genuinely hope that the information and insights provided within these pages have enriched your understanding and will guide you in your journey towards improved health and well-being.

If you found value in this book, would you be so kind as to share your thoughts in a quick review? To write a few words about what you liked, what you learned, or how you plan to apply this knowledge, would be immensely appreciated. Please use the QR code below:

Thank you once again for your time, your curiosity, and your desire to learn. It has been a privilege to accompany you on this journey.

To your health and well-being,

Julia E. Chatwin

Julia E. Chatwin

About the Author

Julia Chatwin is an independent consultant and researcher. Her passion for a scientific approach to health and well-being is the driving force behind her literary contributions, manifesting in a desire to both deepen her own understanding, and enlighten others. An experienced author, Julia's prior success is exemplified by her bestselling books "DASH Diet for Beginners" and "Red Light Therapy".

When not working or writing, Julia loves spending time with her family, cooking (especially baking), and walking her Jack Russell Terrier, called Tommy.

More Books by Julia E. Chatwin

If you enjoyed this book, you may also be interested in the author's other books:

DASH Diet for Beginners

Embark on a transformative journey towards optimal health with "DASH Diet for Beginners". This comprehensive guide, backed by science, unravels the intricacies of the DASH diet in an easily digestible format perfect for beginners. Dive deep into the basic principles of the DASH diet and cook delicious DASH-friendly meals. Full of practical tips and evidence-based advice.

<ins>Available from Amazon</ins>

Red Light Therapy

This book explores the science behind red light therapy, its benefits, how it works, and how you can incorporate it into your daily routine to improve your health and well-being. Whether you are a curious newcomer or a seasoned practitioner, this book will provide you with the knowledge and tools to take advantage of the many benefits that red light therapy has to offer.

<ins>Available from Amazon</ins>

Bibliography and References

The following sources and references have guided and supported the creation of this book. Here, you will find academic research papers, scientific studies, reputable websites, and other relevant publications. I encourage you to explore these references further, delve deeper into specific topics, and gain a better perspective on the landscape of DASH and exercise beyond the confines of this book.

American Heart Association. (2018). *How much sodium should I eat per day?* Www.heart.org. https://www.heart.org/en/healthy-living/healthy-eating/eat-smart/sodium/how-much-sodium-should-i-eat-per-day

Appel, L. J., Moore, T. J., Obarzanek, E., Vollmer, W. M., Svetkey, L. P., Sacks, F. M., Bray, G. A., Vogt, T. M., Cutler, J. A., Windhauser, M. M., Lin, P.-H., Karanja, N., Simons-Morton, D., McCullough, M., Swain, J., Steele, P., Evans, M. A., Miller, E. R., & Harsha, D. W. (1997). A Clinical Trial of the Effects of Dietary Patterns on Blood Pressure. *New England Journal of Medicine*, *336*(16), 1117–1124. https://doi.org/10.1056/nejm199704173361601

Blumenthal, J. A. (2010). Effects of the DASH Diet Alone and in Combination With Exercise and Weight Loss on Blood Pressure and Cardiovascular Biomarkers in Men and Women With High Blood Pressure. *Archives of Internal Medicine*, *170*(2), 126. https://doi.org/10.1001/archinternmed.2009.470

"Body Weight Planner | NIDDK." *www.niddk.nih.gov*, www.niddk.nih.gov/bwp.

Boston, 677 Huntington Avenue, and Ma 02115 +1495-1000. "Sleep." *Obesity Prevention Source*, 21 Oct. 2012, www.hsph.harvard.edu/obesity-prevention-source/obesity-

causes/sleep-and-
obesity/#:~:text=Waking%20Up%20to%20Sleep.

Brown, J. D., Buscemi, J., Milsom, V., Malcolm, R., & O'Neil, P. M. (2015). Effects on cardiovascular risk factors of weight losses limited to 5–10 %. *Translational Behavioral Medicine, 6*(3), 339–346. https://doi.org/10.1007/s13142-015-0353-9

Centers of Disease Control and Prevention. (n.d.-a). *Benefits of physical activity.* U.S. Department of Health and Human Services. https://www.cdc.gov/physicalactivity/basics/pa-health/index.htm

Centers for Disease Control and Prevention. (n.d.-b). *Physical activity for a healthy weight.* U.S. Department of Health and Human Services. https://www.cdc.gov/healthyweight/physical_activity/index.html

Eckel, R. H., Jakicic, J. M., Ard, J. D., de Jesus, J. M., Miller, N. H., Hubbard, V. S., Lee, I-Min., Lichtenstein, A. H., Loria, C. M., Millen, B. E., Nonas, C. A., Sacks, F. M., Smith, S. C., Svetkey, L. P., Wadden, T. A., & Yanovski, S. Z. (2013). 2013 AHA/ACC Guideline on Lifestyle Management to Reduce Cardiovascular Risk. *Circulation, 129*(25 suppl 2), S76–S99. https://doi.org/10.1161/01.cir.0000437740.48606.d1

"Following the DASH Eating Plan | NHLBI, NIH." *Www.nhlbi.nih.gov*, www.nhlbi.nih.gov/education/dash/following-dash.

"Food High in Carbohydrate - NutriVals." *Www.nutrivals.com*, www.nutrivals.com/nutrients/macronutrients/carbohydrate/. Accessed 11 Aug. 2023.

GET THE FACTS. (2017). https://www.cdc.gov/salt/pdfs/sodium_dietary_guidelines.pdf

Gunnars, Kris. "Intermittent Fasting 101 — the Ultimate Beginner's Guide." *Healthline*, 20 Apr. 2020, www.healthline.com/nutrition/intermittent-fasting-guide

Gunnars, Kris. "How Protein Can Help You Lose Weight Naturally." *Healthline*, Healthline Media, 29 May 2017, www.healthline.com/nutrition/how-protein-can-help-you-lose-weight.

Guo, R., Li, N., Yang, R., Liao, X.-Y., Zhang, Y., Zhu, B.-F., Zhao, Q., Chen, L., Zhang, Y.-G., & Lei, Y. (2021). Effects of the Modified DASH Diet on Adults With Elevated Blood Pressure or Hypertension: A Systematic Review and Meta-Analysis. Frontiers in Nutrition, 8. https://doi.org/10.3389/fnut.2021.725020

Hall, K. D., Sacks, G., Chandramohan, D., Chow, C. C., Wang, Y. C., Gortmaker, S. L., & Swinburn, B. A. (2011). Quantification of the effect of energy imbalance on bodyweight. *The Lancet*, *378*(9793), 826–837. https://doi.org/10.1016/s0140-6736(11)60812-x

Harvard Health Publishing. "The Health Benefits of Tai Chi." *Harvard Health*, Harvard Health, 20 Aug. 2019, www.health.harvard.edu/staying-healthy/the-health-benefits-of-tai-chi.

"High Blood Pressure." *CRCHC*, www.crchc.org/high-blood-pressure.

"How Much Is Healthy Weight Loss per Month - Nao Medical." *Naomedical.com*, naomedical.com/info/how-much-is-healthy-weight-loss-per-month.html. Accessed 11 Aug. 2023.

How to Lose 5 Pounds in a Week - Health Lab. 11 June 2023, healthfirstlab.com/how-to-lose-5-pounds-in-a-week/. Accessed 11 Aug. 2023.

Johnston, Carol S. "Strategies for Healthy Weight Loss: From Vitamin c to the Glycemic Response." *Journal of the American College of Nutrition*, vol. 24, no. 3, 1 June 2005, pp. 158–165, pubmed.ncbi.nlm.nih.gov/15930480/, https://doi.org/10.1080/07315724.2005.10719460.

Kapil, V., Khambata, R. S., Robertson, A., Caulfield, M. J., & Ahluwalia, A. (2015). Dietary Nitrate Provides Sustained Blood Pressure Lowering in Hypertensive Patients. *Hypertension*, *65*(2), 320–327. https://doi.org/10.1161/hypertensionaha.114.04675

Kerr, M. (2012). *Exercise and Weight Loss: Importance, Benefits & Examples.* Healthline. https://www.healthline.com/health/exercise-and-weight-loss

Kim, H., Appel, L. J., Lichtenstein, A. H., Wong, K. E., Chatterjee, N., Rhee, E. P., & Rebholz, C. M. (2023). *Metabolomic Profiles Associated With Blood Pressure Reduction in Response to the DASH and DASH-Sodium Dietary Interventions.* https://doi.org/10.1161/hypertensionaha.123.20901

Lim, Eun-Ju, and Eun-Jung Hyun. "The Impacts of Pilates and Yoga on Health-Promoting Behaviors and Subjective Health Status." *International Journal of Environmental Research and Public Health*, vol. 18, no. 7, 6 Apr. 2021, p. 3802, https://doi.org/10.3390/ijerph18073802.

Malacoff, J. (2021, April 9). *10 fitness and weight loss myths trainers want you to stop believing.* InStyle. https://www.instyle.com/beauty/health-fitness/fitness-weight-loss-myths

Mandolesi, L., Polverino, A., Montuori, S., Foti, F., Ferraioli, G., Sorrentino, P., & Sorrentino, G. (2018). Effects of physical exercise on cognitive functioning and wellbeing: Biological and psychological benefits. *Frontiers in Psychology*, *9*(9). https://doi.org/10.3389/fpsyg.2018.00509

Mayo Clinic. "DASH Diet: Guide to Recommended Servings." *Mayo Clinic*, 2019, www.mayoclinic.org/healthy-lifestyle/nutrition-and-healthy-eating/in-depth/dash-diet/art-20050989.

Mayo Clinic. (2021, June 25). *DASH diet: Healthy Eating to Lower Your Blood Pressure.* Mayo Clinic. https://www.mayoclinic.org/healthy-lifestyle/nutrition-and-healthy-eating/in-depth/dash-diet/art-20048456

MHA. "The Best Diet to Lose 10 Pounds Quickly." *Medical Health Authority*, 4 July 2023, medicalhealthauthority.com/health/best-diet-lose-10-pounds-quickly/. Accessed 11 Aug. 2023.

Moore, S. C., Lee, I-Min., Weiderpass, E., Campbell, P. T., Sampson, J. N., Kitahara, C. M., Keadle, S. K., Arem, H., Berrington de Gonzalez, A., Hartge, P., Adami, H.-O., Blair, C. K., Borch, K. B., Boyd, E., Check, D. P., Fournier, A., Freedman, N. D., Gunter, M., Johannson, M., & Khaw, K.-T. (2016). Association of Leisure-Time Physical Activity With Risk of 26 Types of Cancer in 1.44 Million Adults. *JAMA Internal Medicine, 176*(6), 816–825. https://doi.org/10.1001/jamainternmed.2016.1548

NIH. (2021). *DASH Eating Plan | NHLBI, NIH*. Nih.gov. https://www.nhlbi.nih.gov/education/dash-eating-plan

Onodihan. "Effective Strategies for Successful Weight Loss." *Medium*, 22 May 2023, medium.com/@onodihan/effective-strategies-for-successful-weight-loss-5693cfc33868. Accessed 10 Aug. 2023.

Schiavon, C. A., Bersch-Ferreira, A. C., Santucci, E. V., Oliveira, J. D., Torreglosa, C. R., Bueno, P. T., Frayha, J. C., Santos, R. N., Damiani, L. P., Noujaim, P. M., Halpern, H., Monteiro, F. L. J., Cohen, R. V., Uchoa, C. H., de Souza, M. G., Amodeo, C., Bortolotto, L., Ikeoka, D., Drager, L. F., & Cavalcanti, A. B. (2018). Effects of Bariatric Surgery in Obese Patients With Hypertension. *Circulation, 137*(11), 1132–1142. https://doi.org/10.1161/circulationaha.117.032130

Soltani, S., Shirani, F., Chitsazi, M. J., & Salehi-Abargouei, A. (2016). The effect of dietary approaches to stop hypertension (DASH) diet on weight and body composition in adults: a systematic review and meta-analysis of randomized controlled clinical trials. Obesity reviews: an official journal of the International Association for the

Study of Obesity, 17(5), 442–454.
https://doi.org/10.1111/obr.12391

West, Helen. "The Complete Beginner's Guide to the DASH Diet."
Healthline, Healthline Media, 17 Oct. 2018,
www.healthline.com/nutrition/dash-diet.

Woodyard, Catherine. "Exploring the Therapeutic Effects of Yoga and Its
Ability to Increase Quality of Life." *International Journal of Yoga*, vol.
4, no. 2, 2011, pp. 49–54,
www.ncbi.nlm.nih.gov/pmc/articles/PMC3193654/,
https://doi.org/10.4103/0973-6131.85485.

Made in the USA
Las Vegas, NV
02 January 2024

83805403R00132